Stop for a moment and think about the person you love most. It may be a child, perhaps a wife, partner or husband, maybe your sister or brother. Now imagine fate intervening, and this special person suffers a stroke, traumatic brain injury, or other form of acquired brain injury. Those who survive come back to the land of the living, but irrevocably changed as persons – different from the person whom the relative fell in love with. Most academic textbooks fail to capture the effects that the tragedy of acquired brain injury has on those around the patient – the relatives. *Family Experience of Brain Injury: Surviving, Coping, Adjusting* does not. Through the powerful narratives of relatives telling their unique stories, and commentaries by professionals, the lifelong journey of grief, loss, compassion and hope that families go through is vividly told. While this is a book primarily intended for those working with families after brain injury, all clinicians, academics and researchers working in the field of neurorehabilitation should read this book.

Dr Rudi Coetzer, Consultant Neuropsychologist and
Head of Service, North Wales Brain Injury Service,
Betsi Cadwaladr University Health Board, NHS Wales, UK

Family Experience of Brain Injury

Brain injury not only affects its victim, but those around them. In many cases, relatives are often overlooked despite facing many obstacles accepting and adjusting to a new way of life. *Family Experience of Brain Injury* showcases a unique collaboration between relatives of brain injured individuals and professionals from the field of neuro-rehabilitation. Family members from all different viewpoints tell their story and how the brain injury of a loved one has affected them.

This book provides a space for those hidden and marginalised voices, the people who are in for the long haul, often dismissed by services and left to cope in isolation. By combining expert commentary with real life experiences, this book points towards sources of support, normalises the experience and provides a context for understanding the grief and losses of family members. Not only will the hard-earned knowledge and wisdom evident in this book help educate health and social care staff, but it highlights how love, commitment, hope and perseverance, against a seemingly unbearable grief, can remain.

It is essential reading for individuals and families touched by brain injury and will give multi-disciplinary professionals, such as medics, nurses, psychologists, therapists, social workers, rehabilitation practitioners and clinical supervisors, a greater understanding of their role in helping the affected family.

Jo Clark-Wilson qualified as an Occupational Therapist in 1979, then studied with the Open University to complete a degree in psychology and research. She has had the privilege of working with individuals with brain injury and their families for the past 30 years.

Mark Holloway By accident Mark became a support worker for people with brain injuries nearly 30 years ago; he qualified as a social worker in 1995 and continues to work with individuals and families affected by brain injury.

After Brain Injury: Survivor Stories

Series Editor: Barbara A. Wilson

This new series of books is aimed at those who have suffered a brain injury, and their families and carers. Each book focuses on a different condition, such as face blindness, amnesia and neglect, or diagnosis, such as encephalitis and locked-in syndrome, resulting from brain injury. Readers will learn about life before the brain injury, the early days of diagnosis, the effects of the brain injury, the process of rehabilitation, and life now. Alongside this personal perspective, professional commentary is also provided by a specialist in neuropsychological rehabilitation, making the books relevant for professionals working in rehabilitation such as psychologists, speech and language therapists, occupational therapists, social workers and rehabilitation doctors. They will also appeal to clinical psychology trainees and undergraduate and graduate students in neuropsychology, rehabilitation science, and related courses who value the case study approach.

With this series, we also hope to help expand awareness of brain injury and its consequences. The World Health Organisation has recently acknowledged the need to raise the profile of mental health issues (with the WHO Mental Health Action Plan 2013-20) and we believe there needs to be a similar focus on psychological, neurological and behavioural issues caused by brain disorder, and a deeper understanding of the importance of rehabilitation support. Giving a voice to these survivors of brain injury is a step in the right direction.

Locked-In Syndrome After Brain Damage
Living Within My Head
Barbara A. Wilson, Paul Allen, Anita Rose, and Veronika Kubickova

Rebuilding Life after Brain Injury
Dreamtalk
Sheena McDonald, Allan Little, Gail Robinson

Family Experience of Brain Injury
Surviving, Coping, Adjusting
Jo Clark-Wilson and Mark Holloway

For more information about this series, please visit: https://www.routledge.com/After-Brain-Injury-Survivor-Stories/book-series/ABI.

Family Experience of Brain Injury

Surviving, Coping, Adjusting

Jo Clark-Wilson and Mark Holloway

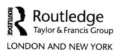
Routledge
Taylor & Francis Group

LONDON AND NEW YORK

First published 2020
by Routledge
2 Park Square, Milton Park, Abingdon, Oxon OX14 4RN

and by Routledge
52 Vanderbilt Avenue, New York, NY 10017

Routledge is an imprint of the Taylor & Francis Group, an informa business

British Library Cataloguing in Publication Data
A catalogue record for this book is available from the British Library

Library of Congress Cataloging-in-Publication Data
A catalog record has been requested for this book

ISBN: 978-1-138-89666-6 (hbk)
ISBN: 978-1-138-89669-7 (pbk)
ISBN: 978-1-315-17906-3 (ebk)

Typeset in Times New Roman
by Taylor & Francis Books

Contents

List of boxes   viii
Acknowledgements   ix
Foreword   x
Preface   xiv

1   Introduction   1

2   Acquired brain injury and families: The context   3

3   Does the family become part of the team, or the team
become part of the family?: An interview with a father 17
years after brain injury   22

4   Behaviour, vulnerability and the criminal justice system   44

5   Grief without end   60

6   Support of siblings   77

7   Children's challenges   92

8   The impact of acquired brain injury on the family:
Common themes, threads and differences   113

9   What may help?   138

10   In conclusion   158

References   162
Index   169

Boxes

6.1 Professional reflection: relationships with family 81
6.2 Professional reflection: differences in outlook 82
6.3 Professional reflection: ambiguous loss 88
6.4 Professional reflections: meaning of life 89
7.1 Professional reflection: need for safety and immediate support 100
7.2 Professional reflection: safeguarding 101
7.3 Professional reflection: discrepancies 104
7.4 Professional reflection: knowledge is power 111

Acknowledgements

We would like to acknowledge all those families that have enabled us to learn from their experiences over time, as this has allowed us to develop greater understanding of what might help others to cope, survive and even flourish after brain injury. To them we owe a lifetime of gratitude.

We would also like to thank Dr Doreen Baxter, for her review of our work and help in the writing of the book; and Janine Heritage and the staff at Head First, who have provided ongoing support and encouragement.

Foreword

This book written by Jo Clark-Wilson and Mark Holloway provides an in-depth insight into the experiences of family members whose loved ones have experienced a brain injury. The book covers their experiences from the point of injury and throughout their lifetimes in detailed and compassionate accounts reflected on by brain injury specialists working with them and their family members. Working with the person with the brain injury to ensure life-long integration is an important part of the work of a range of community specialists, including, but not limited to case managers. But what is often not addressed is the importance of working with families as well as the individuals themselves.[1]

Throughout the book the authors introduce the reader to characters with important stories to tell. We meet Dan, whose son Paul was injured when he was hit by a car at the age of 15 years; Jeanne, whose son Adam was injured in a road traffic accident when he was 21 years old; and Laura, whose husband had a stroke at age 50. Other accounts include those of Eliza and Grace who both have siblings with brain injuries; and Alistair, Beatrix and Deirdre who have parents with a brain injury. While professionals often focus on the needs of the individual with the brain injury, the effects of the injury do not occur in isolation. Instead the impact of that injury is far reaching and touches the lives of everyone close to that individual. While everyone's story is different, this book highlights key themes that run throughout the accounts: trauma, ambiguous loss, the burden of care and a sense of being alone.

Chapters 4 and 7 particularly emphasise the impact of the initial trauma on family members. After the incident, family members wait anxiously by their loved one's bedside hoping that they will pull through. This is encapsulated within the narratives, alongside the 'hindsight' reflection of whether they had wished for the right outcome. That early hope when someone wakes from a coma is often short-lived as the reality of the situation they are facing begins to take hold. Many of the accounts mentioned examples of people pointing out how 'lucky' they were that their loved ones were alive or looked 'normal'. Deirdre reflected on this in Chapter 7 when she describes that looking back at the road traffic accident that killed her mother and injured her father, the worst possible outcome would have been both her parents surviving with a brain injury. This is a contentious issue and one that family members may feel unable to discuss with others who do not understand the grief that they are experiencing, or their ongoing hardship.

Chapter 3 provides a striking account of Dan's grief at having nearly 'lost' his son in a road traffic accident and his ongoing sense of ambiguous loss, a theme that runs throughout the accounts. Ambiguous loss refers to the sense of grieving for a person who may be physically present but is psychologically no longer the same.[2] For many family members ambiguous loss is often at the fore. The personality, behavioural, cognitive and executive impairments experienced by individuals with brain injuries often fundamentally changes who they are as a person, which makes it difficult for their loved ones to accept. The true 'essence' of the person has been lost. Families have to struggle with the position of continuing to live and support their loved one who is physically present while managing their internal sense of grief for the person who is no longer in their lives.

As well as the trauma of the initial event, there are all the subsequent traumas that often go unnoticed by professionals and friends, even extended family members. The accounts talk of behavioural issues, poor decision-making, drinking too heavily, getting into trouble with the police, abusive actions, and so on. These are the day-to-day traumas experienced by family members – not intense life-changing traumas but a drip feed effect of constantly living on high alert, wondering when the next incident will occur, when the next phone call or knock on the door might come. This reality does not come to an end – they are in it for a lifetime. This, mixed with ambiguous loss, leaves family members feeling trapped and helpless, a factor well known to be associated with mental health problems, especially depression.[3] Day-to-day life for family members is exhausting.

Chapter 3 also describes the importance of how the relationship between the case manager and the family develops. While not all families necessarily have their loved one's 'best interests' at heart, most do, and their experience of the incident and the ongoing injury is as important as the client's. They are a fount of knowledge about the person in terms of understanding pre-morbidity and changes post-injury.

They are also bereaved and traumatised and therefore in need of a safe space where they can support their loved one. The book highlights the good practice of case managers who are matched based on shared values with clients and their families but who also do not shy away from awkward situations and possible aggression from family members. Instead they hold fast and listen to the family and try to understand their perspective. This is a principle that is important, not just for case managers, but for all professionals working with individuals with brain injuries and their families. It is important to listen, and even more important to hear, to ensure that the needs of families are reflected, their views and experience acknowledged, and any misunderstandings rectified early on. This good practice is contrasted with many of the accounts in this book that emphasise the often poor knowledge professionals have of brain injury, but also a lack of compassion and empathy, and inability to 'come alongside' the client and their family. Instead the professionals either provide nothing in the way of support, or make wrongful assumptions about the reasons for behaviours (such as laziness), or assumptions that the person is less disabled than they are. Assumptions are made about the family – that they are overprotective and interfering – leading to them being dismissed and ignored. The account of Laura in Chapter 5 also raises the issue of the burden professionals place on family members – almost an assumption that they should and will look after their loved ones even if they have immense needs, have changed fundamentally as people, and the family member still has other responsibilities to uphold.

The various perspectives taken in the book highlight the impact of brain injury on all the family. It is not just the primary caregiver who may suffer – it is the siblings, the children, the step-parents. The stories touch upon the complexities of managing brain injury within the family context where there may already be conflicts and hardships that have to be overcome alongside the consequences of the brain injury. They also touch upon the consequences of brain injury, not just for the individual but for family members too; such as a 17-year-old teenage girl who witnesses her brother nearly dying in front of her and then goes on to support his rehabilitation, neglecting her own needs and developing deep-seated psychological issues as a consequence; such as the 8-year-old boy who loses his friends and develops an unhealthy relationship with food because he feels neglect due to his mother's time being focused on his older brother who now needs round-the-clock care. The book also emphasises the differences in the experiences of each individual, not just in terms of their role in the loved one's life, but also in terms of where they happened to be, or what they happened to experience, at the time of the initial incident. These differing perspectives are often forgotten in the chaos of the daily grind of managing brain injury. However, taking the time to process and understand is important for preventing rifts within families or future difficulties in family dynamics, or to resolve fundamental misunderstandings – like that of an 8-year-old who assumes that his brother is dead.

This book is a must read for professionals and family members alike. The accounts within it provide comfort and support to family members and remind them that they are not alone. For professionals, the book provides some important lessons. There is too much focus on the individual with the brain injury and not enough on the family as a wider unit. Family therapy and support is fundamental to the process of adjustment and should not be viewed as an unnecessary luxury. It is fundamental to the family's ability to function and paramount in enabling them to support the needs of their loved one. Family members also need to feel part of the process. They may not understand complex medical jargon, or feel comfortable in highly formalised medical settings, such as multidisciplinary team meetings – they may need advocacy to make their perspective heard, and support to advocate for their loved one. Finally, the book emphasises the importance of ongoing community support for the person with the brain injury – brain injury has life-long consequences and a life-long approach must be adopted to rehabilitation and care.

Dr Alyson Norman

Notes

1 Horwitz, R.C., Horwitz, S.H., Orsini, J., Antoine, R.L., & Hill, D.M. 1998. Including families in collaborative care: impact on recovery. *Journal of Families, Systems and Health*, 16, 71.
2 Boss, P. 2006. *Loss, trauma, and resilience: therapeutic work with ambiguous loss*. New York and London: W.W. Norton.
3 Miller, W.R., & Seligman, M.E. 1975. Depression and learned helplessness in man. *Journal of Abnormal Psychology*, 84, 228–238.

Preface

We must free ourselves of the hope that the sea will ever rest. We must learn to sail in high winds.

(Aristotle Onassis)

Owing to advances in medical care and improvements in the practice of neurorehabilitation (in countries where such services are available), today many more people across the world are surviving an acquired brain injury. Increasingly the stories of brain injured people feature in books and on social media; their battles back from the very brink of death to meaningful if altered lives are told – sometimes humorously, but always movingly. The sister books in this series stand as wonderful proof of the power of bearing witness to the testimony of survivors, each story so very different and yet with a common thread; a life unexpectedly altered in an instant.

Having worked with people affected by brain injury for many decades, we would argue brain injuries do not just occur to just the injured individual, but also to those people around them. This is a story of loved ones and families whose lives are affected, sometimes very significantly. These individuals, the people who work tirelessly to support their injured family members often without adequate support (or any support at all in some cases), have stories to tell. Their trauma, their Sisyphean experiences of endless love in the context of unending grief, is often missed if the focus remains only upon the injured party (if upon any party at all). We believe that such individuals are also survivors, not only indirectly but directly too, surviving the experience of loss and grief for what was but can never be again; survivors of the services and the society that they are left to navigate in their newly acquired and unwelcomed status as 'relative of a person with a brain injury'.

This book has been written with parents, spouses, children and siblings, who have been supporting their relative after brain injury for long periods of time. Three family members, a mother, a father and a spouse, with direct and long-standing experience of acquired brain injury have each written their story in this book, describing their experiences and providing us with the wisdom they had never hoped to gain. Each of these people has been paired up with a specialist from the professional 'world of brain injury' who provides a commentary on their story. One of the authors, Jo Clark-Wilson, gives voice to those relatives whose stories are pushed even further to the periphery, the children and siblings of brain injured people, and Jo reflects on her own professional practice and personal learning over the decades.

Whilst each of our family members tells a different and unique story, there are some common themes that develop and it may be useful to consider those in the context of research aimed at describing the relative's experience (Holloway, 2017). In this research, in common with what is described in this book, family members describe how the context of the accident has an impact as to how this is experienced and felt by them and their injured relative. The nature of such injuries affects all aspects of the non-injured party's life and leads to their inevitable involvement in myriad tasks, from basic day-to-day management and practical support, to behavioural and emotional support and liaison with outside individuals/authorities. Family members' experience of formal and informal support structures impacts upon their experience, their grief and losses, which in turn affects their involvement with the injured party. Overarching this is the theme of the relative being the only party who holds the injured person's life-history together in a cogent way. The family member becomes the curator of the narrative of their loved one.

Just as this book is written from a number of different perspectives, we hope that its readership will also be broad-based, offering ideas and information to both family members and professionals, be they long in the tooth (like us) or in training and about to embark upon their careers.

As will be seen in the pages that follow, family members often report that their voices are not heard, that their individual stories remain untold, that they are not helped and the potential benefit of their wisdom and hard-won knowledge is ignored. For this reason, we expressly gave permission for the family members and professionals that they were paired with to tell the story as they saw fit; we have not edited their work to match our aims but have left their words in their voice. This may make for some uncomfortable reading for our professional audience: themes of poor treatment (or of no treatment) by services are repeated and the genuine grief experienced by family members is at times very raw. For this we make absolutely no apology, indeed quite the reverse, for since family members state clearly that integrating them, their knowledge and their experience is what is required, we must surely start with hearing the words that they use. If their grief is too difficult to hear, what must it be like to live? Do we as professionals avert our eyes and our ears on occasion because the act of listening properly would remind us of our own fragility?

Each of our family members describes the experience of having a loved one suffer a severe brain injury, one which has changed them too. At points their stories are despairing, at other points they demonstrate resilience and hope, but most of all they demonstrate enduring and relentless love. Each family member agreed to participate because they wanted their experience to help others, to help professionals understand and improve their practice but, perhaps more importantly, to provide other affected family members with the strength and courage to continue loving in the face of unimaginable adversity. For this we owe them a great debt of gratitude. Their stories are not over of course. If you are a professional holding this book in your hands, you can choose whether you put this book down or not. In providing their loved ones' care, they do not have the privilege of such choices.

If you are a family member affected by brain injury, we hope that the insights and information contained within help support you to manage your story. The book finishes with a chapter on suggestions for what may work to help support you.

You are not alone.

If you are a professional, either one well versed in all the long-term complexities of brain injury and with many years of experience or new to the condition, we also hope that the insights and information contained within this book support you to understand more about the experience and role of family members, why their role is key and why they require support. You too are not alone.

Recovery from severe brain injury is a long road for all concerned; each journey must begin with that first step.

References

Holloway, M. 2017. Acquired brain injury: the lived experience of family members. Doctoral thesis, DSW, University of Sussex.

Onassis. 2001. *Brainy Quote.* https://www.brainyquote.com/quotes/aristotle_onassis_119069.

Chapter 1

Introduction

The impact of severe brain injury is complex, far-reaching and extremely challenging. The range of difficulties reported as a consequence of the injury, both in terms of impairments and their functional impact, were noted by all contributors in this book to have caused very significant changes to their relative's lives and potential future options.

In this book, we start by considering the underlying issues of brain injury and describe what can occur after this type of trauma. We describe the process of rehabilitation, the potential professionals involved and changes over time in different settings. There will be a review of research articles on functional outcomes over time, highlighting those on brain injury and family functioning.

We then introduce each of our contributors, i.e. father and mother, spouse, siblings and children, all of whom have their own unique relationship, not only with the individual who has sustained the brain injury but with all other members of the family, who have also been traumatised by the impact of the same incident. They have provided their own unique stories; a description of their relative who sustained the brain injury and a narrative of their experiences since this trauma occurred. The majority of these family members provide reflections after supporting their relative for long periods of time, in some cases over 25 years, and they have valuable advice to offer for others in similar situations.

It was evident many of the behavioural changes caused by the brain injury made the care and support of their relative extremely difficult. Risks associated with poor executive functioning, lack of insight and empathy, unpredictability and impulsiveness, and social vulnerability were noted to be challenging and, in these situations, often no clear resolutions could be found. Some of our contributors still provide high levels of care and support, and continue to be under prolonged stress, often without respite.

Professionals, who have been working in the field of brain injury for long periods of time, each provide reflections and comments on one or more of the contributions.

The relatives' narratives are reviewed in detail, looking at common threads and themes shared by other contributors. These themes also explored the nature of the overall functioning of the family unit, including extended family, over time, and over different generations. There has also been further investigation of their roles as parent, spouse, child or sibling, to establish if there are any issues arising from their stories that are unique to that specific role.

These common threads and themes, and the recommendations as given by the contributors, are then reviewed in the context of the current literature to see what can be done in the future to support families of individuals with severe brain injury.

Chapter 2

Acquired brain injury and families
The context

As people, we all have different personalities, values, skills and abilities. Our unique and individual experience of life shapes what we do and how we view things. To a greater or lesser extent, we have set routines, structured roles and responsibilities within our family unit, acting within the norms of our community, culture and society. Within families there are complex patterns of interactions, interconnections and emotional interdependencies, all of which are unique and special to that individual family member and group. Shared experiences and expectations shape how we cope and support each other throughout the ups and downs of life. Facing or dealing with issues together provides us with a sense of safety, security and stability.

Acquired Brain Injury (ABI) can occur to anyone, anytime, within our family, work and social networks. You will know people who have sustained an injury – but you may not be aware of it, as many of the difficulties associated with ABI are not visible. In this chapter we look briefly at the impact of ABI upon an individual, the role of rehabilitation services in recovery from and adaptation to the condition, and look at the impact this has upon family members.

Brain injury

Brain injuries happen as a consequence of a trauma of some kind, such as a road traffic accident or assault, or can be caused by myriad other issues such as encephalitis, loss of oxygen to the brain or a stroke. Whatever the cause, a brain injury is often sudden and unexpected, and the impact can be life changing. The consequences of damage to the brain are always unique for that individual.

Brain injury can result in complex presentations of fatigue, pain, sensory and physical impairments, language difficulties, cognitive and emotional disorders, and personality changes. Slowness in processing information, difficulties in concentration, recalling information, problem-solving and decision-making; and behaviour changes, for instance, irritability, impulsivity, rigidity of thinking, unpredictability, social disinhibition and aggression, may all be subtle (or not so subtle) signs of a brain injury.

Deficits are often 'invisible' and all impact on everyday functioning, social integration and restoration of the individual's previous 'normal' lifestyle. Outcomes are very difficult to predict, as many factors can affect recovery and the individual's opportunities to progress and re-establish their life. Sister books in this Survivors' Stories series provide excellent examples of how individuals can thrive following a brain injury, how improvements to life and quality of life are possible, at least for some. Those excellent examples, however, also give testimony to just how difficult this can be, and just how long this can take.

Due to incredible medical advances over the past 30 years, more people are surviving a brain injury than previously. Unfortunately, these improvements in acute medical treatment are not matched by adequate provision of the post-injury rehabilitation and the support required to improve these survivors' return to independence, occupation and social activities, or enhance their quality of life. Family members are often key in facilitating a quality of life for their relative with a brain injury, by playing a central role in providing support and care, as well as advocating on behalf of their loved one.

Acquired brain injury: the impact

Floyd Skloot, an American poet and novelist, who wrote about his search for meaning of personal loss after experiencing encephalitis, noted:

> I used to be able to think. My brain's circuits were all connected, and I had spark, a quickness of mind that let me function well in the world. I could reason and total up numbers; I could find the right word, could hold a thought in mind, match faces with names, converse coherently in crowded hallways, learn new tasks. I had a memory and an intuition that I could trust.
>
> (Skloot, 2003, p. 3)

And

> brain injury intensifies the meaning of sudden personal change by affecting the very organ with which we define who we are. The brain, where mind and body come together, where Self originates,

is transformed in an instant. Not just how we see or speak, how we feel or think, what we know or recall, but who we are is no longer the same. Without warning, without choice we are Other.

(Skloot, 2003, p. ix)

As we progress through childhood into adulthood, guidance from older adults tends to diminish as we gain skills, become competent at tasks and learn to manage our environment better (Jackson and Hague, 2013). Routines, and an ability to maintain our goals and direct our behaviour mean that we tend to become increasingly self-reliant. The effects and outcomes of a brain injury vary considerably but dealing with life-threatening trauma, having significant changes to self and increased dependency affects not only the individual with brain injury but also their family and friends. There are some issues that present particular challenges for family members.

Invisible changes

Carroll and Coetzer found individuals with brain injury in their study reported significant changes in self-concept. Their present-self was viewed negatively in comparison to their pre-injury self. The greater the individual's perception of identity change was, the greater the likelihood of reported depression and grief (Carroll and Coetzer, 2011). Higher levels of awareness are also associated with poorer self-esteem (Cooper-Evans et al., 2008). Fleminger et al. (2003) suggested vulnerability to depression and suicide by the person with the ABI might relate to psychological factors, such as the recognition of losses (Fleminger et al., 2003).

Invisible deficits create most challenges, as people (even many professionals) do not recognise that how the individual with the brain injury presents is not always a true reflection of their abilities.

If a person presents with a broken leg, everyone can see it as well as the related medical interventions and treatments, and people are also over time, able to witness progress and recovery.

(Fleminger and Ponsford, 2005)

'Executive' problems

Some people are noted to suffer 'executive impairments' following an ABI and these can create difficulties in formulating goals, planning and problem solving, and effectively carrying out plans. When a person has difficulties in formulating a plan towards a goal then they may react impulsively or respond to their environment without regard for the consequences.

Disorders of executive functioning are not always easily discernible in immediate conversations, particularly in a highly structured conversation, but become notable over time in everyday decision making and behaviours. It has been reported that everyday decision making does not take place 'in the head'; it takes place '*in the world*' and this involves navigating a decision, a situation which is populated with options, opportunities, dangers and temptations (Owen et al., 2017). Family members therefore may be more aware of these invisible difficulties than professionals. Family members see changes over a longer time period and have 'pre-brain injury' experience to compare to post-brain injury behaviour or actions.

Specialists working in the field of acquired brain injury recognise the need for assessments of individuals to take place over time and within the context of their environment. Listening to family members and relevant others, in addition to the individual with brain injury, is crucial for a realistic perspective of the situation in order to fully appreciate the individual and their family's needs.

Insight

Floyd Skloot is able to personally reflect and express the changes created by his brain injury, whereas many people, as a consequence of the damage caused by their trauma, are unable to do this. People who have sustained severe injuries, particularly to the frontal and pre-frontal areas of the brain, are not always able to easily make adaptations, and many lack awareness or insight into their condition. According to Crosson et al., the person does

> not realise that a problem is occurring therefore they do not recognise the need to initiate compensation. It is only afterwards, when someone else has pointed out the problem or the patient has reasoned through the unexpected results, that he or she can recognise what was happening.
>
> (Crosson et al., 1989)

Having awareness of their condition is not the same as insight. In clinical practice some people will have awareness of their difficulty when this is pointed out to them but demonstrate an inability to use this information when faced with the same or similar situations in the real world. Again, it is the family member, who may be best placed to see this difference between what someone says they can do/will do and what actually happens in reality.

In reality family members and professionals are often faced with the real challenge that the person with the brain injury does not see things the way others may do. It is very hard to support someone or encourage them to get help if they do not think there is a problem. Challenging a person's viewpoint can be counter-productive and cause an individual not to engage with the very services and support that may help them. Family members may find themselves in the very difficult situation of having a relative who does not see that they have a problem trying to access services that, similarly, fail to pick up on the invisible difficulties that brain injury may bring.

People with executive deficits and poor insight have an increased vulnerability within this 'real world'. The impact of the brain injury on their ability to monitor their behaviour, to self-regulate and correct mistakes causes ongoing and repeated 'disinhibited' behaviours. Many patients with frontal lobe injuries are described as 'childish', 'lazy', 'insensitive' and/or 'aggressive'. They can have difficulty checking or modifying their basic feelings and drive, leading to repeated socially inappropriate behaviours, e.g. gaining large amounts of weight, drinking to excess, or becoming grossly indiscriminate in their approach to sexual partners (Jackson and Hague, 2013). People with traumatic brain injury who exhibit behaviour that is verbally or physically aggressive, socially inappropriate or sexually disinhibited often find themselves socially isolated from their peers after brain injury (Kozloff, 1987). The inability to identify social cues and delay (or inhibit) action when aroused often contributes to poor choices. This, when also seen in the context of being unable to appreciate other people's points of view or demonstrate empathy for others, has devastating social consequences.

These difficulties often lead to increasing social isolation. The associated vulnerability can lead an individual to seek the company of people who may exploit them, as the brain injured individual is unable to read their intentions. There is often clear evidence from families that the person is unable to function in the real world, is at risk and is in need of services, as they have an increased dependency on the environment.

Executive dysfunction and traumatic brain injury are noted as significant variables in offending behaviour; a systematic review of research showed the prevalence of traumatic brain injury among incarcerated youths ranged from 49 per cent to 72 per cent. This was also linked to earlier, repeated offences, greater time in custody and more violent offending (Williams et al., 2015).

Recovery and rehabilitation

The journey from the accident and emergency department to (a degree of) acceptance and adjustment following a life changing injury or illness is a long one; both for the injured party and for their family.

Floyd Skloot wrote of his experience when considering the need to accept the changes in himself:

> Acceptance is a deceptive word. It suggests a compliance, a consenting to my condition and to who I have become. This form of acceptance is often seen as weakness, submission. We say, 'I accept my punishment.' Or 'I accept your decision.' But such assent, while passive in essence, does not provide the stable, rocklike foundation for coping with a condition that will not go away.
>
> (Skloot, 2004, p. 197)

He went on to note that:

> Such shifts of value made possible by active acceptance of life as it is, can only be achieved alone. Doctors, therapists, rehabilitation professionals, family members, friends, lovers cannot reconcile a person to the changes wrought by illness or injury, though they can ease the way. Acceptance is a private act, achieved gradually and with little outward evidence. It also seems never to be complete ... But for all its private essence, acceptance cannot be expressed purely in private terms. My experience did not happen to me alone; family, colleagues and friends, acquaintances were all involved.
>
> (Skloot, 2004, p. 198)

In the early stages of recovery, the acute treatment in hospital concentrates on the medical and nursing care. Family members visit and support relatives during their emergence from coma into the disoriented, confused, distressed and agitated state of the 'post-traumatic amnesia' phase. Therapy is focused upon physical impairments, communication and functional routines, as this enables the individual with brain injury to feel better, move around and express their wishes, and have increased independence in simple everyday tasks (Trevena-Peters et al., 2018).

Discharge planning from hospital can be difficult to manage. For those individuals who are unable to return home, in the UK there are very few residential neurorehabilitation units suitable for people with brain injury. Even when a placement is available the injured individual often has to stay some distance away from family and friends.

The individual with the brain injury may return home before they and their family recognise or are ready to deal with the changes that have occurred. Family members quickly have to learn how to care for, rehabilitate and support their changed, disoriented, and traumatised relative. This can place extreme demands and undue stress on the family, as they may have to provide 24-hour care without a full appreciation of their relative's problems or needs. On many occasions this care is given without information or guidance on how to care and support their relative, backup support or rehabilitation services.

A number of models of rehabilitation after severe brain injury have been identified (Clark-Wilson et al., 2014, Wilson et al., 2009), and these approaches facilitate different styles of learning to enhance greater independence. Rehabilitation following brain injury ideally moves from predictable, structured tasks towards more complex, less structured situations, as it is discovered how the individual best copes and what can be achieved to enable them to function more independently. In many cases it is helpful for families to be involved in supporting their relatives generalise work from rehabilitation settings, into the individual's daily environments, in order to maximise the potential of any learning achieved during the rehabilitation process.

'Invisible deficits' (cognitive, emotional and behavioural) usually become more evident over time. Cognitive and personality changes after brain injury gradually become revealed as the individual participates in more complex, unstructured situations. If the community places too great a demand upon the individual, perhaps because they are too chaotic and unpredictable, rehabilitation may need to take place in a setting where a therapeutic milieu is more controlled and demands upon an individual are more easily managed.

Responding to change is cognitively demanding at any time, but for an individual after brain injury this can be particularly difficult. Re-establishing self-identity and self-confidence, and adapting and developing new routines, roles and relationships can be extremely challenging.

If the patient does not experience, at some level, the usefulness of the rehabilitation programme, he or she will resist treatment or only passively engage in it. Thus, the first principle of neuropsychological rehabilitation is that the clinician must enter the patient's phenomenological field in order to sense what he or she experiences. The reality of helping patients not to be alone with their disturbances and helping them to deal with their disordered experience is of maximum value.

(Prigitano, 1999, pp. 28–29)

Gracey and Ownsworth noted the first relationship the injured person has to make is the new relationship with him/herself. They describe how the individual's adjustment before and after injury is one of comparisons, judgements and evaluations, considering their past self, present or idealised self and future self. Finding an identity following changes after a severe brain injury is even harder for individuals who have sustained their injury at a young age, before they know who they are. Identity is mixed up within a social context (Gracey and Ownsworth, 2008). Identity is not just about who we think we are, but also who others think we are (Jenkins, 2006). Finding a place in the real world within the family is both cognitively and emotionally changing. It requires a degree of abstract thought. The very skills one needs to do this may be damaged by the brain injury.

If, as is hoped, the individual with brain injury develops greater independence in everyday skills, they will experience greater autonomy and reduced direction from others involved in the rehabilitation and support process. Nevertheless they may still have significant life changes to deal with. Reduced abilities, significant losses, such as increased isolation from social contacts, and uncertainties about the future, create an emotional and psychological impact that can lead to depression, anxiety and even suicidal thoughts. This is not only the case for the individual with the brain injury but also for family members, who may gradually have less support from those professionals experienced in brain injury that might be able to help them. They may also be in the position where they have to provide continued support for their injured relative.

Statutory health and social care services in the UK are stretched and have limited resources to meet the diverse and unique issues presented by brain injury. Services operate within parameters that do not necessarily match up with the difficulties presented by this condition. Few professionals working in statutory services have specialist experience in working with this particular client group over time and this creates many issues for individuals and their families. Under-resourced professionals are likely to identify their own goals and outcomes for the injured individual rather than spend their limited time supporting families or developing shared goals and involving them closely in the design of rehabilitation interventions. An absence of adequate resources for specialist rehabilitation services means that family members not only have to care for their relative but also to actively seek their own support.

Lack of expertise in brain injury was also identified by the House of Lords Select Committee when scrutinising the Mental Capacity Act in 2014. It was noted they received a number of submissions from professionals working with individuals who had sustained a brain injury, who expressed concern about whether those without experience in this field were able to correctly assess mental capacity. This submission from the British Association of Brain Injury Case Managers (BABICM) illustrates the point:

> Clients who have a good residual intellect, who present plausibly and articulate their thoughts well are likely to be considered to have capacity to manage their own affairs, even despite a lengthy history of impulsivity, lack of social judgement, tangential thought processes, problems with attention and a lack of insight into how their cognitive deficits affect their decision making. Yet this is a client group who can still be extremely vulnerable to malign influence and coercion, particularly if they are in possession of a lump sum of money.
>
> (Acquired Brain Injury and Mental Capacity Act
> Interest Group, 2014, p. 29)

Further training (or perhaps any training) would enable professionals to recognise and understand the issues, so they can hear what family members say rather than just take what the injured person says at face value. Taking the time to be available for people with a brain injury and their families (at the time when it is most needed) can reduce the trauma felt by individuals and family members. This was the case for families interviewed by Mark Holloway, who also considered specialist brain injury case managers were the most helpful professional group in supporting them over time.

After brain injury, every individual embarks on their own journey and, over time, the reality of their circumstances becomes evident. The family can be integral to how positive outcomes can be achieved. It may involve promoting increased independence, resuming family life with the roles they had previously, spending time with friends, or a return to some form of structured, purposeful occupation and social lifestyle. Or, in cases where this is not possible, this may be about improving quality of life. The encouragement and consistent support of family members provides the support and determination the injured person needs to keep moving forwards to reach their goals.

Family and brain injury

The makeup and functioning of families varies considerably, culturally and within a single family across time, and there is a sense of interdependence between family members (as well as independence from each other) (Covey, 2014).

Members of families (parent, spouse, child, sibling, grandparents) may take on specific roles and responsibilities for the functioning of the family unit. These roles are sometimes clearly defined and explicit, for instance, provision of physical resources (wage earner); nurturing and emotional support for other family members; childcare and social educator; the making of decisions; or sharing of family household roles, like cooking dinner, managing finances or doing/organising repairs. Other roles are unique, according to the personalities involved, their life experiences, and their perceptions of sensitivities and needs of other family members. Stronger family functioning is observed when individual family members know their responsibilities and subtly adapt these over time, as they are required to support and maintain the changing family unit. The family member's role is always expanding or changing over time as children grow, parents age, and so on.

When a family member acquires a brain injury, it not only affects the individual concerned, it will also greatly impact upon the family as a social group. The nature of this impact on any family and family member is unique and varies enormously. Family members have their own narrative, as they are often left to struggle with understanding the changes that have occurred to their relative, and to learn and develop ways to adapt to a new and different way of life consequent to this trauma.

Family and brain injury research

The stories told by relatives in this book can be set into the context of what this research teaches us. First and foremost, after a brain injury, relatives are thrust into the unfamiliar territories of the emergency room, acute care and, possibly, rehabilitation services. Nobody is prepared for this. To make matters worse, the majority of people with a brain injury are discharged home to the family for their care, often within a short period of time and without adequate support (Blake, 2014). Family members are therefore unprepared for what is going to happen and yet are left to be responsible. When we compare that to another great challenge experienced by families, that of becoming a parent, we can see stark differences. People are usually aware that they will become a parent, most of us have family members or friends who are parents who can share their experience and wisdom, and there is much advice and support available to help us understand what the role entails and what to expect. This is not the case with brain injury. The challenge may be huge but the formal and informal support available may be very limited.

When individuals sustain a severe brain injury, the family may cling desperately to the hope of 'a miracle', particularly in the early stages of recovery. Their wait is often a lengthy one, full of uncertainty, which may lead families to postpone and delegate usual responsibilities, again leading to feeling guilty for leaving chores and other family members with unmet needs (Lefebvre et al., 2007). It is not possible for a family member to be in two places at once after all, and the injured person may, understandably, take priority.

Research into the impact of acquired brain injury upon family members has identified significant levels of stress and burden upon relatives. The stories our relatives tell in this book mirror this research. Our authors tell of the difficulties they have faced but they tell of more than this; they speak of their resilience, the lessons they have learnt over time, and of a strength that they did not previously know that they had. Perhaps by understanding a little more about the research and listening more to what family members say, professional staff may be better placed to recognise the role of family and understand what supports them best? Understanding what the issues are and what works seems like a good place to start.

Levels of burden and stress vary amongst family members; not everyone has the same experience, of course. The impact of burden and stress upon family/carers is identified as being a risk for the development of psychiatric and other health difficulties (Moules and Chandler, 1999). The burden experienced is greater than that for carers of people with other conditions (Jackson et al., 2009) and carers report having needs unmet by adequate service provision (Blake, 2014). Carer burden is noted to increase over time and not to level out or lessen (Levor and Jansen, 2000, Jordan and Linden, 2013).

Stress, as a result of trauma, can lead to sleep disturbances, loss of appetite, difficulties in concentrating, anger and rage, anxiety, fear and terror, shame, grief, disassociation and ruminations. Stress can result from an experienced single traumatic event or develop, as the complexity of traumatic experiences becomes so overwhelming that the individual can no longer maintain their resilience. Cognitive, emotional and behavioural changes in the person with ABI are noted to be the strongest predictor of clinically significant anxiety and depression for family members and of unhealthy family functioning (Ponsford et al., 2003). These are the 'invisible difficulties' others find hard to understand but relatives generally see more clearly.

The nature of the trauma experienced by family is one where the security provided by the assumptive world can be lost, and previously held beliefs about, and for the future are shattered (Kauffman, 2002). Unlike bereavement, the nature of this loss is ambiguous as the injured party is physically present, alive, and yet altered. The person's personality is potentially so changed as to be unrecognisable in some instances, more subtly changed in others. The very nature of the condition itself may prevent the injured party from understanding or accepting that they have changed. The individual may also have potentially lost the capacity to empathise or pay attention to the needs of others too.

It is this ambiguity of the losses felt that separates ABI from many other traumatic events. The injured person may look the same, sound the same and even think that they are the same as before the brain injury, but it is the relative who sees the changes. Boss defined ambiguity in this context as a lack of clarity as follows:

> When the adjective ambiguous is used to describe a loss, it means there is no validation or clarification of the loss, and thus a lack of knowing whether the lost person is irretrievably lost or coming back again.
>
> (Boss, 2006)

Such ambiguous loss is identified as unresolved grief (Boss, 1999a), as there is no 'closure' and acceptance is made impossible because the loss is ongoing (Boss and Carnes, 2012). Put most simply, there is no body to bury, and no culturally accepted ceremonies to support the 'non-bereaved' as there are with death. Life goes on but grief remains 'frozen' (Boss, 1999b) as the ambiguity and the loss experienced combine to create an obstacle to coping and grieving (Boss, 2006). Family members are noted to lack a 'road-map' (Jordan and Linden, 2013). The experience is described as:

a lifelong journey of understanding disabilities and impairment while working to accept the changes that have occurred in one's life. Caregivers embark on a parallel journey of coming to terms with a 'new normal' as the person they once knew is forever changed due to the brain injury.

(Petersen and Sanders, 2015)

Boss and others note that this ambiguity experienced by family members produces ambivalence, a sense of conflicting (potentially entirely contradictory) emotions (Boss, 2010). These feelings of ambivalence can be so severe as for parents of brain-injured people to both love and wish their children dead at the same time (Webb, 1998). Such ambivalence, when set in the context of invisibility of impairment and a brain-injured relative who lacks insight into their condition – who can neither empathise nor be grateful for the support they receive – places family members under extreme stress (Ergh et al., 2002). Lack of support from the wider community, and attitudes to people with an ABI can compound these difficulties (Linden and Boylan, 2010) whereas increased resilience of family members is noted to correlate with positive outcomes in relation to family well-being (Simpson and Jones, 2013).

There are unique relationships, whether that of parent, spouse, sibling or child, and research has investigated some of these.

Studies that have looked at the relationship between adults with an ABI and their parents (Kao and Stuifbergen, 2004, Knox et al., 2016, Jones and Morris, 2013, Wongvatunyu and Porter, 2008a, Wongvatunyu and Porter, 2008b) have focussed upon the change in the relationship between the parents and their children, the parents' concerns about the reduced independence of their child and, unsurprisingly, longer-term concerns about what would happen when they were unavailable to provide support.

In respect to spouses or partners, relationship breakdown has been noted to be high in some studies (Wood and Yurdakul, 1997). However, in surviving relationships, significant changes occur in role, identity, security and loss of previously held future options and beliefs change the relationship greatly (Godwin et al., 2014). Sexual health and behaviour are negatively affected for many (Simpson and Baguley, 2012, Simpson et al., 2013).

Loss of relationships and friendships are common (Rowlands, 2000, Prigatano and Gupta, 2006) and affected by such issues as varied as facial recognition ability (Knox and Douglas, 2009), loss of conversational abilities (Shorland and Douglas, 2010) and alexithymia (difficulties in emotional awareness, social attachment, and inter-personal relating) (Williams and Wood, 2013). Literature focusing on supporting relationships post-injury is frequently based around notions of improving communication and communicational abilities (Togher et al., 2016, Togher, 2013, Murphy et al., 2015), and improving functional outcome by changing the approach undertaken by the non-injured party in particular.

Siblings may be disregarded, yet the sibling relationships are the ones that may last the longest. Siblings may take over the caring or support roles from parents after the parents are unable to continue in this role. The impact upon siblings, including adult siblings with or without a formal care role, is not well investigated (Degeneffe, 2016, Degeneffe, 2015, Degeneffe and Olney, 2010).

The children of people with an ABI are noted to be negatively affected, for instance 48 per cent of children in one study found to suffer symptoms of Post Traumatic Stress Disorder (PTSD) (Kieffer-Kristensen et al., 2011), and are at higher risk of emotional and behavioural difficulties (Butera-Prinzi and Perlesz, 2004, Uysal et al., 1998). Skilled and specialised social work and brain injury case management intervention has been identified as effective in helping parents with an ABI to support their children (Holloway and Tyrrell, 2016).

The literature relating to childhood ABI contains work with an emphasis on identifying and supporting behavioural change by parents to support the engagement with and management of children with an ABI, as well as the impact felt by their parents. Interventions to improve parenting abilities are identified (Brown et al., 2015, Brown et al., 2014), some focused on parent coping style (Prihadi et al., 2015) and others upon supporting return to education (Andersson et al., 2016). The direct impact upon parents was identified as being significant (De Kloet et al., 2015, Heary et al., 2004).

Conclusion

It is clear that the role of a family member of a person with an ABI is not an enviable one. The difficulties experienced are exacer-bated by a lack of understanding of the condition by the wider community and by severely under-funded rehabilitation and support services. Family members are therefore left with few options but to provide support for the person with an ABI. Despite these very real difficulties, and as demonstrated in the following chapters, there is reason for optimism.

References

Acquired Brain Injury and Mental Capacity Act Interest Group 2014. *Making the abstract real: recommendations for action following the House of Lords Select Committee Post-Legislative Scrutiny Report into the Mental Capacity Act.* In: www.babicm.org/uploads/doh-mca-abi-17-09-14.pdf (ed.). London.

Andersson, K., Bellon, M., & Walker, R. 2016. Parents' experiences of their child's return to school following acquired brain injury (ABI): a systematic review of qualitative studies. *Brain Injury,* 30, 829–838.

Blake, H. 2014. Caregiver stress in traumatic brain injury. *International Journal of Therapy and Rehabilitation,* 15, 263–271.

Boss, P. 1999a. *Ambiguous loss: learning to live with unresolved grief.* Cambridge, MA and London: Harvard University Press.

Boss, P. 1999b. Insights: ambiguous loss: living with frozen grief. *The Harvard Mental Health Letter from Harvard Medical School,* 16, 4–6.

Boss, P. 2000. *Ambiguous loss.* Cambridge, MA: Harvard University Press.

Boss, P. 2006. *Loss, trauma and resilience: therapeutic work with ambiguous loss.* New York: W.W. Norton.

Boss, P. 2010. The trauma and complicated grief of ambiguous loss. *Pastoral Psychology,* 59, 137–145.

Boss, P., & Carnes, D. 2012. The myth of closure. *Family Process,* 51, 456–469.

Brooks, D.N., & McKinlay, W. 1983. Personality and behavioural change after severe blunt head injury: a relative's view. *J Neurol Neurosurg Psychiatry,* 46, 336–344.

Brooks, N. 1991. The head-injured family. *Journal of Clinical and Experimental Neuropsychology,* 13, 155–188.

Brown, F. L., Whittingham, K., Boyd, R.N., Mckinlay, L., & Sofronoff, K. 2014. Improving child and parenting outcomes following paediatric acquired brain injury: a randomised controlled trial of Stepping Stones Triple P plus Acceptance and Commitment Therapy. *J Child Psychol Psychiatry Allied Discip,* 55, 1172–1183.

Brown, F.L., Whittingham, K., Boyd, R.N., Mckinlay, L., & Sofronoff, K. 2015. Does Stepping Stones Triple P plus Acceptance and Commitment Therapy improve parent, couple, and family adjustment following paediatric acquired brain injury? A randomised controlled trial. *Behav Res Ther,* 73, 58–66.

Butera-Prinzi, F., & Perlesz, A. 2004. Through children's eyes: children's experience of living with a parent with an acquired brain injury. *Brain Injury,* 18, 83–101.

Caroll, E., & Coetzer, R. 2011. Identity, grief and self-awareness after traumatic brain injury. *Neuropsychological Rehabilitation,* 21(3), 289–305.

Clark-Wilson, J., Giles, G.M., & Baxter, D.M. 2014. Revisiting the neurofunctional approach: conceptualizing the core components for the rehabilitation of everyday living skills. *Brain Injury,* 28(13–14), 1646–1656.

Cooper Evans, S., Alderman, N., Knight, C., & Oddy, M. 2008. Self-esteem as a predictor of psychological distress after severe acquired brain injury: an exploratory study. *Neuropsychological Rehabilitation,* 18(5), 607–626.

Covey, S.R. 2014. *The 7 habits of highly effective families.* New York: St. Martin's Press.

Crosson, B., Barco, P.P., Velozo, C.A., Bolesta, M.M., Cooper, P., Werts, D., & Brobeck, T.C. 1989. Awareness and compensation in postacute head injury rehabilitation. *Journal of Head Trauma Rehabilitation,* 4, 46–54.

De Kloet, A.J., Lambregts, S.A.M., Berger, M.A.M., Van Markus, F., Wolterbeek, R., & Vliet Vlieland, T.P.M. 2015. Family impact of acquired brain injury in children and youth. *Journal of Developmental and Behavioral Pediatrics,* 36, 342–351.

Degeneffe, C.E. 2015. Planning for an uncertain future: sibling and parent perspectives on future caregiving for persons with acquired brain injury. *Journal of Rehabilitation,* 81, 5–16.

Degeneffe, C.E. 2016. A clarion call for social work attention: brothers and sisters of persons with acquired brain injury in the United States. *Journal of Social Work in Disability and Rehabilitation,* 1–18.

Degeneffe, C.E, & Olney, M.F. 2010. 'We are the forgotten victims': perspectives of adult siblings of persons with traumatic brain injury. *Brain Injury,* 24 (12), 1416–1427.

Ergh, T.C., Rapport, L.J., Coleman, R.D., & Hanks, R.A. 2002. Predictors of caregiver and family functioning following traumatic brain injury: social support moderates caregiver distress. *Journal of Head Trauma Rehabilitation,* 17, 155–174.

Fleminger, S., Oliver, D.L., Williams, W., and Evans, J. 2003. The neuropsychiatry of depression after brain injury. *Neuropsychological Rehabilitation,* 13(1–2), 65–87.

Fleminger, S., & Ponsford, J. 2005. Long term outcome after traumatic brain injury. *British Medical Journal,* 331, 1419–1420.

Godwin, E., Chappell, B., & Kreutzer, J. 2014. Relationships after TBI: a grounded research study. *Brain Injury,* 28, 398–413.

Gracey, F., & Ownsworth, T. (eds) 2008. The self and identity in rehabilitation. *Neuropsychological Rehabilitation* (Special Issue), 18(5–6).

Heary, C., Hogan, D., & Smyth, C. 2004. Parenting a child with acquired brain injury: a qualitative study. *Psychology and Health,* 19, 74–75.

Holloway, M., & Tyrrell, L. 2016. Acquired brain injury, parenting, social work and rehabilitation: supporting parents to support their children. *Journal of Social Work in Disability and Rehabilitation,* 15(3–4), 234–259.

Jackson, D., Turner-Stokes, L., Murray, J., Leese, M., & Mcpherson, K.M. 2009. Acquired brain injury and dementia: a comparison of carer experiences. *Brain Injury,* 23, 433–444.

Jackson, H.F., & Hague, G. 2013. Social consequences and social solutions: community neurorehabilitation in real social environments. In: *Practical neuropsychological rehabilitation in acquired brain injury* (Newby, G., Coetzer, R. & Daisley, A., eds). London: Karnac Books.

Jenkins, R. 2006. *Social identity.* Abingdon: Routledge.

Jones, L., & Morris, R. 2013. Experiences of adult stroke survivors and their parent carers: a qualitative study. *Clinical Rehabilitation,* 27, 272–280.

Jordan, J., & Linden, M.A. 2013. 'It's like a problem that doesn't exist': the emotional well-being of mothers caring for a child with brain injury. *Brain Injury*, 27, 1063–1072.

Kao, H.F., & Stuifbergen, A.K. 2004. Love and load: the lived experience of the mother–child relationship among young adult traumatic brain-injured survivors. *Journal of the American Association of Neuroscience Nurses*, 36, 73–81.

Kauffman, J. 2002. *Loss of the assumptive world: a theory of traumatic loss.* New York and London: Brunner-Routledge.

Kieffer-Kristensen, R., Teasdale, T.W., & Bilenberg, N. 2011. Post-traumatic stress symptoms and psychological functioning in children of parents with acquired brain injury. *Brain Injury*, 25, 752–760.

Knox, L., & Douglas, J. 2009. Long-term ability to interpret facial expression after traumatic brain injury and its relation to social integration. *Brain and Cognition*, 69, 442–449.

Knox, L., Douglas, J.M., & Bigby, C. 2016. 'I won't be around forever': understanding the decision-making experiences of adults with severe TBI and their parents. *Neuropsychological Rehabilitation*, 26, 236–260.

Kozloff, R. 1987. Network of social support and the outcome from severe head injury. *Journal of Head Trauma Rehabilitation*, 2, 14–23.

Lefebvre, H., Pelchat, D., & Levert, M. 2007. Interdisciplinary family intervention program: A partnership among health professionals, traumatic brain injury patients and care giving relatives. *Journal of Trauma Nursing*, 14, 100–113.

Levor, K.D., & Jansen, P. 2000. The traumatic onset of disabling injury in a marriage partner: self-reports of the experience by able-bodied spouses. *Social Work*, 36, 193–201.

Linden, M.A., & Boylan, A.M. 2010. 'To be accepted as normal': public understanding and misconceptions concerning survivors of brain injury. *Brain Injury*, 24, 642–650.

Moules, S., & Chandler, B.J. 1999. A study of the health and social needs of carers of traumatically brain injured individuals served by one community rehabilitation team. *Brain Injury*, 13, 983–993.

Murphy, A., Huang, H., Montgomery, E.B.Jr., & Turkstra, L. 2015. Conversational turn-taking in adults with acquired brain injury. *Aphasiology*, 29, 151–168.

Owen, G.S., Freyenhagen, F., Martin, W., & David, A.S. 2017. Clinical assessment of decision-making capacity in acquired brain injury with personality change. *Neuropsychological rehabilitation*, 27, 133–148.

Petersen, H., & Sanders, S. 2015. Caregiving and traumatic brain injury: coping with grief and loss. *Health and Social Work*, 40, 325–328. doi:10.1093/hsw/hlv063.

Piccenna, L., Lannin, N.A., Gruen, R., Pattuwage, L., & Bragge, P. 2016. The experience of discharge for patients with an acquired brain injury from the inpatient to the community setting: a qualitative review. *Brain Injury*, 30, 241–251.

Ponsford, J., Olver, J., Ponsford, M., & Nelms, R. 2003. Long-term adjustment of families following traumatic brain injury where comprehensive rehabilitation has been provided. *Brain Injury*, 17, 453–468.

Prigitano, G.P. 1999. *Principles of neuropsychological rehabilitation*. Oxford: Oxford University Press.

Prigatano, G.P., & Gupta, S. 2006. Friends after traumatic brain injury in children. *Journal of Head Trauma Rehabilitation*, 21, 505–513.

Prihadi, E.J., Dings, F., & Van Heugten, C.M. 2015. Coping styles of parents of children and adolescents with acquired brain injury in the chronic phase. *J Rehabil Med*, 47, 210–215.

Rowlands, A. 2000. Understanding social support and friendship: implications for intervention after acquired brain injury. *Brain Impairment*, 1.

Shorland, J., & Douglas, J.M. 2010. Understanding the role of communication in maintaining and forming friendships following traumatic brain injury. *Brain Injury*, 24, 569–580.

Simpson, G., & Jones, K. 2013. How important is resilience among family members supporting relatives with traumatic brain injury or spinal cord injury? *Clinical Rehabilitation*, 27, 367–377.

Simpson, G., Sabaz, M., & Daher, M. 2013. Prevalence, clinical features, and correlates of inappropriate sexual behavior after traumatic brain injury: a multicenter study. *Journal of Head Trauma Rehabilitation*, 28, 202–210.

Simpson, G.K., & Baguley, I.J. 2012. Prevalence, correlates, mechanisms, and treatment of sexual health problems after traumatic brain injury: a scoping review. *Critical Reviews in Physical and Rehabilitation Medicine*, 24, 1–34.

Sinnakaruppan, I., & Williams, D.M. 2001. Family carers and the adult head-injured: a critical review of carers' needs. *Brain Injury*, 15, 653–672.

Skloot, F. 2004. *In the shadow of memory*. Lincoln, NE: University of Nebraska Press.

Togher, L. 2013. Improving communication for people with brain injury in the 21st century: the value of collaboration. *Brain Impairment*, 14, 130–138.

Togher, L., Mcdonald, S., Tate, R., Rietdijk, R., & Power, E. 2016. The effectiveness of social communication partner training for adults with severe chronic TBI and their families using a measure of perceived communication ability. *NeuroRehabilitation*, 38, 243–255.

Trevena-Peters, J., Ponsford, J., & McKay, A. 2018. Agitated behavior and activities of daily living retraining during posttraumatic amnesia. *The Journal of Head Trauma Rehabilitation*, 33(5), 317–325.

Uysal, S., Hibbard, M.R., Robillard, D., Pappadopulos, E., & Jaffe, M. 1998. The effect of parental traumatic brain injury on parenting and child behavior. *Journal of Head Trauma Rehabilitation*, 13, 57–71.

Webb, D. 1998. A 'revenge' on modern times: notes on traumatic brain injury. *Sociology*, 32, 541–555.

Williams, C., & Wood, R.L. 2013. The impact of alexithymia on relationship quality and satisfaction following traumatic brain injury. *Journal of Head Trauma Rehabilitation*, 28, E21–E30.

Williams, H., Hughes, N., Williams, W., Chitsabesan, P., Walesby, R.C., Mounce, L.T., & Clasby, B.J. 2015. The prevalence of traumatic brain injury among young offenders in custody: a systematic review. *Journal of Head Trauma Rehabilitation*, 30, 94–105.

Wilson, B.A., Gracey, F., Malley, D., Bateman, A., & Evans, J.J. 2009. The Oliver Zangwill Centre approach to neuropsychological rehabilitation. In: idem, *Neuropsychological Rehabilitation: Theory, Models, Therapy*. Cambridge: Cambridge University Press.

Wongvatunyu, S., & Porter, E.J. 2008a. Changes in family life perceived by mothers of young adult TBI survivors. *Journal of Family Nursing*, 14, 314–332.

Wongvatunyu, S., & Porter, E.J. 2008b. Helping young adult children with traumatic brain injury: the life-world of mothers. *Qualitative Health Research*, 18, 1062–1074.

Wood, R.L., & Yurdakul, L.K. 1997. Change in relationship status following traumatic brain injury. *Brain Injury*, 11, 491–501.

Chapter 3

Does the family become part of the team, or the team become part of the family?

An interview with a father 17 years after brain injury

This chapter is based on the interviews of Dr Siobhan Palmer, Consultant Neuropsychologist with Dan, Paul's dad.

Introduction

I first met Dan in a coffee shop when he was talking with his son's case manager, who introduced us. If I had asked Dan for a description of the values that he lives his life by, I imagine he would have respectfully replied that he doesn't have time to think about that, but 'just cracks on'. To me, the listener, Dan seems strong; a person driven by loyalty and respect, but mostly by love for his family. Dan is a man who stands up for himself and his family above everything else. His family values are so deeply rooted that he does not even recognise them as values or his life compass, he simply is as he is.

He tells me that before his son's injury, his own emotions were raw and unfiltered. Yet, after the injury, Dan had to learn how to fight without his fists, to negotiate a world of polite conversation and trust people who he didn't always believe.

As the result of a collision whilst crossing the road, Dan's son Paul has profound (yet invisible) cognitive impairments. Fully mobile, without obvious scarring or communication problems, Paul's inability to initiate *anything* prevented him from managing his basic needs without an extensive care package. Dan described some of his memories of how he needed to fight to give his son the support he needed. As with many individuals after brain injury, the invisibility of his cognitive impairment led to conflicting opinions within the medico-legal context and vastly different recommendations for long term support needs, which was confusing and frustrating for Dan and his family. Sadly, not an unfamiliar story. They learned that within a structured, routine environment, Paul could function relatively well but outside of that environment he neglected himself. Remarkably, when he was asked to paint a room 'starting with this wall' he willingly set about painting the one wall and then stopped. He was found standing in the room, looking a little lost, unable to work out what to do next. He had taken the starting instruction literally and, unable to problem solve, he didn't finish painting the room but instead stood for hours awaiting the return of his voluntary work employer to give the next instruction. On another occasion, the opposite problem happened: once started he didn't stop ... his mother asked him to decorate the stairs and banisters. His intention had been to sand and then paint them. He started sanding but couldn't work out when it was time to stop sanding and move onto the next stage of undercoating. So, he sanded excessively and returned home with blisters across his hands.

Dan describes in a matter of fact way that his commitment to his children is lifelong, or for as long as they need him. Dan has negotiated dilemmas about when to give autonomy, when to support and when to make decisions on Paul's behalf. He was granted power of attorney and, together with his wife, has made many decisions around complex issues such as contraception, housing, parenting and relationships, which required him to navigate the (now less foreign) world of solicitors, courts and lengthy paperwork. Paul is now married with two children and lives a happy, settled (routine) life.

In this chapter, Dan describes his experience of fighting for Paul's disability to be recognised, his own battles along the way, and how things are now, 17 years later. I am struck by Dan's composure and calmness in describing his experience of disenfranchised grief; a loss but yet not. A son who is still here and shows no recognition of having been lost. The invisibility of Paul's issues means Dan and his family still need to trawl over the evidence and present it to professionals each time someone new comes into Paul's life, to help Paul access this and that. The disability is not obvious for others to see, but hard for Dan to see past sometimes. It creates tough battles, especially in this unfamiliar world of solicitors, case managers, professionals and people who seem to speak a different language. In fighting those battles, Dan has discovered abilities he did not know he had; patience, tolerance and eloquence. It's bitter sweet that his unremitting dedication to help his son ('whatever it takes') has meant improving his own communication skills, and these have probably improved his life outside of Paul's care.

We met twice in a cafe, drinking tea. The first time, I mostly listened to his conversation with the case manager. The second time, armed with questions and a dictaphone, I tried to find out more about how the relationship with the case manager had done a complete U-turn. Dan's thoughts flowed naturally and engagingly, with humour, sadness and humility. I am reminded of how important it is for people to tell their story and for it to be recognised and validated. I listen intently, recognising that whilst there are overlaps in this story and in those of other relatives, I have never heard this story before. It is a great responsibility to represent this in the right way for Dan. Dan has been honest enough to sit in a cafe with tears in his eyes, wanting his message of patience, listening and personal connection to be heard, so the message can go on and help other families out there. We met a final time, and that time I really started to get it; this is not Dan's story, or Paul's story, but the story of how a young family united. Initially they united *in spite of* the brain injury, but perhaps more latterly they became stronger and closer *because of* the brain injury.

I outline our interviews, with much of the text transcribed verbatim.

Conversation

Tell me a bit about you

I'm Paul's Dad. I was brought up in a challenging family environment in the 1960s through the 1970s, as one of five children with an additional six step brothers and sisters. Being one of eleven doesn't mean you were not loved, but it does mean family was a big part of my life. There was just one breadwinner (our step father) and our mother stayed at home looking after us. The way children were brought up in those days was different to how we brought our children up in the 1980s, 1990s and through the millennium. I grew up on a council estate and had the life that went with it (life was different on a council estate in those days). I have worked in the construction industry for all but five years of my adult life. I don't consider myself academic, as I left school with no qualifications. I fell in and out of jobs for a few years then had children and thought I had better settle down and ensure that they were looked after.

Family is important to me. I have four children. At the time of Paul's injury I was living in a two-room flat with my wife (Anna) and our two young children (Luke, aged 2 and Grace, aged 2 weeks). We also lived with my older boys Paul (15) and John (13). We had been happily living there for a couple of years.

Can you give me a description of how your life is with Paul now?

It's hard to answer this, as life with Paul now is lots of different normal things, like anybody's life with their adult child, but there is a tension inside me about whether to grieve or be proud. You have those feelings together at the same time. I can give you a real example of our life these days. My wife and I popped in to a supermarket one sunny day in the summer of 2016; as we walked in we saw two of our granddaughters who were seven and six at the time, with their mother by the magazine stand. You can always hear the girls long before you see them, loud is an understatement, but endearing. As I looked towards the fresh fruit aisle I saw our eldest son, stood still looking in to space, almost appearing in a trance. I touched him. 'What's up Son?' 'Nothing Dad, just looking for the wife and kids.' 'Over by the magazines.' 'Thanks Dad.' Off he goes to see the girls and his wife, calm and unphased. I am in despair, to me it never ends, there's no getting away from it, no relief, it will never get better. (He still gets lost a lot and stands looking into thin air – it's not perhaps as obvious now, but it is if you know him.) My mind transports me to the sunny afternoon on 13th May 2001. I am putting a light up in the porch when there is a knock on the door. My son's friend tells me 'he has just been hit by a car'. When I got to him, I can remember the blood … but more the cut to his temple sticks in my mind. I remember praying he had not hurt his head, you just know if someone hurts their head it cannot be repaired.

Our son suffered a very serious closed brain injury that day, resulting in five bleeds to the brain with the worst being in his frontal lobe.

Back to life as it is now, 17 years later. Paul and I have a 'father and son' relationship, and my wife Anna is essentially his case manager now. I am recognised by the courts as the commissioner of his care. It has taken us 17 years to get back to the point where we have this father–son relationship. There was a large care package which we had to fight for, and we have gradually removed his support until now Paul works solely with Anna.

I constantly check with Anna how Paul is doing; is he working to his care plan, is he maintaining his routines, is he looking after himself? Paul also rings me almost every day and from those phone calls I can glean from him how he is doing, and if I need to intervene. I spend my life scrutinising his life to ensure that he is playing to his strengths and those close to him are working with him to enable him to be what he desires above all else, 'to be the best Dad he can'. If I am the best dad I can be, then by default Paul will be the best dad he can be.

How did life change after the accident?

When your son wakes up from a coma looks you straight in the eye and asks, 'who are you?' … it's life changing.

This event had an impact on everyone, even down to the 2-week-old baby, who had just arrived in this world when all this was going on. The whole process brought a change in all the family. Anna and I decided that we had to put our own feelings aside and had to include Sandra (Paul's birth mother) even though we didn't actually agree. We've been through a torrid time as a family. Together, we have reached a better point than I could have wished for in terms of Paul's life, happiness and being settled with his own family.

Paul lived with us at the time of his accident. His mother decided she wanted to look after him upon his discharge from hospital, and so he went back to live with her. On reflection, this was the start of conflict insofar as differing opinions in Paul's care needs, and as it turns out, this conflict was to remain in the background for 13 years. There was some confusion about whether Paul could make his own decisions.

Shortly after discharge from hospital, Paul was admitted to a neuro assessment centre for a week. His mother and I were informed that he had made a remarkable recovery and would need no further medical intervention. Paul's mother was happy with the assessment, but I was sceptical ...

Paul lived with his mother for 18 months after that, during which time she retained the services of a lawyer to sue the car driver responsible for Paul's injuries. Paul's mother didn't notice the problems we saw, but she did report that he spent time continually counting fish in the fish tank.

When did you begin to notice the cognitive problems?

Paul turned up at home in February 2003 and asked if he could move back in. We had seen Paul during the previous 18 months but only for short periods. We knew he had changed and was not the same active, adventurous person who had gone out jet skiing and things, prior to the accident, but we had put it down to living with his mother as he had a much more relaxed living regime there. Anna and I live an incredibly structured life, as did Paul when he lived with us. Its funny now, looking back, its like we already lived a 'brain injury friendly' way of life, with all our structure and routines.

Within a couple of days of moving back in, problems started arising which became more concerning by the day; falling asleep at college even though he was getting enough sleep at home. He would be constantly fatigued. Paul would not feel hungry, his personal hygiene lapsed even though he was told to shower. One day we asked Paul to go to the shop for a loaf of Hovis and he came back with nothing ...

we asked why and he said they had no Hovis, and when we asked why he did not get an alternative he just looked blankly at us. He couldn't work out what to do. Over a period of months, as we spent time with him it would become noticeable that he would become agitated, repetitive, vacant, bored and displayed signs of OCD (like counting the fish in the tank). We noticed he seemed confused, he had to be told to do things he would not have to be told to do previously. He had lost all of the confidence and personality he had before. Was he grieving for his loss ... why was he behaving immaturely, we wondered?

Tell me about the professionals you met, and how you first met Richard

Well, after he came home in 2003, he had some outpatient Occupational Therapy (OT) but it didn't seem to be addressing the problems we had noticed. We had been told about Headway while Paul was in hospital, and we read their leaflets to find out a bit more. As we read them it was like we were reading about Paul. We realised he must have a brain injury so we decided to speak to the lawyers to discuss the things we'd noticed, and they arranged a meeting with a case management company. They 'matched' us with a case manager who had interests in tattoos, and camping, which Paul liked. This case manager turned out to be Richard.

The first meeting was like an invasion.

Not only were these professionals coming into our house, telling us what we ought to be doing differently with Paul, but the conflict that I also had at the back of my mind (much harder to articulate, and certainly not tangible) was this sense that maybe I don't know my son now, and although I should know my son better than them ... perhaps I don't. It was a lot of difficult feelings.

Its not a criticism but I didn't like the case manager at all when I first met him. He was an intruder. I have never had any dealings with these types of people (people with degrees and notepads) before. He didn't seem to be getting it. He asked Paul and I about his cognitive impairments. To this day, one of the things I would never do is say something negative about the brain injury in front of Paul. I would be positive about what I could, and if I couldn't be positive then I wouldn't talk about it. So, I didn't go through everything because I won't risk making my son feel bad for the benefit of these lawyers and people. As his Dad, it is more important to me to tell him there is nothing wrong than it is to tell the legal team all the problems I have seen.

The difficulty was that Paul also couldn't tell them his problems. If he was told, 'I think you have made a remarkable recovery from your head injury' he would agree, and if he were then told 'you have lots of ongoing issues following your brain injury' he would also agree … . Paul had no real insight in to his cognitive impairment, as we were beginning to learn. It was really galling when the medico-legal process was happening because he agreed with what anybody said, and they were constructing his reality for him, but it didn't always match with ours.

On the basis of his early assessment, Richard (the case manager) suggested moving Paul into his own accommodation away from us. I was fiercely opposed as he still didn't get it. Everything I was working for (I had been working 27 days a month in order to earn enough to look after my family and be the best father that I could be) was not what I was working for anymore. Richard took it up with the solicitor and described me as overprotective, and said I was dismissive of the idea of moving Paul into his own property, and I may become difficult. The solicitor spoke to me about this, and I was so angry to have been described as overprotective and potentially difficult! Richard didn't seem to understand Paul's problems at all. So, by the time of the next meeting with Richard, I had two choices: do I sack him or try and work with him? At many points in this journey, you seem to have two important choices which will change the course of things. With Richard, the solicitor had told me he is a 'good bloke' and I shouldn't lose him, so I knew I had to say my bit without losing him. I knew I had to do it but I didn't know how I would do it. At our next meeting, I waited patiently for him to sit down, and then began asking him who the **** he was judging my wife and I, and the care we give to our children. A full and frank discussion followed, which allowed us to move forward.

It worked out okay.

Do you think the full and frank discussion with the case manager was a turning point in your relationship?

That was the first time I had ever tried to put my point of view across without shouting or threatening, and Richard didn't walk away. That was a point that strengthened my relationship with him and in the end, I agreed with the solicitor that he was a good bloke.

So, yes, it was a turning point. We had a conversation, I got my opinion across and he realised he had to work with me and couldn't do it without me.

I had to learn to listen to Richard and the team, but it takes time. It's not just about time or just about listening, or space to listen, but what its really about is being heard, and really hearing what's being said to you too. It's about being safe enough in the relationship that you can test it and it does not falter. Richard did not leave after we had the very frank and honest discussion; that was 'make or break'. I certainly learned from that moment; I learned that I can speak my mind without shouting or threatening.

Richard talked to us about why he felt Paul needed to trial living independently, but we were not ready for this step, to let Paul go. I wanted to convert our house and put living quarters in for Paul. Practically, looking back there was no way we could have converted our house, but at that time, Richard could not convince me of that. Richard realised at that meeting that inclusion of the family and gaining their buy-in was critical in rehabilitation. I think we learned from each other.

Was there a therapy team?

Yes, along the way, we met some other brilliant professionals too (psychology and OT). These professionals were part of the team. Looking back, I think of them (and Richard) as part of the family. I miss them. You don't miss professionals, but I miss them. They have always been more than just people doing a job. They were straight talking people who didn't pause and think before they spoke (that was how I knew I could trust them and they didn't have another agenda). We were lucky to have these people on our team. I work well in straight talking relationships. Perhaps that's why it worked well with the OT, psychologist and Richard because they're straight talking too and they spoke to me from their heart. They cared.

I always stood in the doorway during Multi-Disciplinary Team (MDT) meetings, with everyone else sat down, distancing myself from the process, not wanting to accept what was going on. I thought I knew what was best for my son. The case manager used to call at me 'come in and sit down Dan, you're making the place look untidy', but I didn't. I did the same thing for many months and Richard said the same thing until one day I just sat down as part of the group.

Did the team help you understand the cognitive problems?

The case manager introduced us to a neuropsychologist who would be able to meet Paul and help us understand his cognitive impairments.

When I met her she just sucked me in, she had me, this woman just knew stuff. She told us that Paul's cognitive difficulties were so subtle they could easily be missed; although professionals would be able to pick up on the memory deficits and obsessional behaviours, they may miss the decision making and initiation problems. She suggested that some family members may not be able to easily understand the nuances of Paul's hidden deficit, and on top of that is the acceptance of the trauma itself.

So, a professional was telling us that we will not only have to educate family, which as mentioned earlier were already in conflict over the outcomes of Paul's brain injury, but now I was being told that we would have to educate some of the professionals as well. I was amazed.

The OT did not at first understand how much time Anna spent supporting Paul each week. As we saw it, he was one of our children who needed time so he got it; it did not occur to us that Paul would be taking up the amount of time he was. She asked Anna to record all of the time she spent with Paul, and what exactly she was asking him to do. Anna was required to go into detail to enable the OT to understand how much independent support Paul would need. She came back to us and reported that Anna had been casually supporting Paul for 70 hours a week. How could a family be supporting a child for 70 hours per week without realising it?! Parenting is a full-time job and you don't actually log the time you spend with one child against another, as they all get the time they need and you just muddle along.

Overall though, Paul helped me understand. I said 'Paul, I don't really get this memory thing', and he said 'Its like dominoes Dad ... when you put another domino on, one falls off the table ... ' and that's how he feels about his memory ... that he doesn't keep things very long. Where he got that from, I'll never know, but that's how he explained it. To me, that made sense then, that bits of his memory just kept falling away. This boy could walk around without anyone picking up at all that he had a brain injury. You needed to speak to him for at least an hour and have an idea about brain injury before you knew there was anything wrong with him at all. There is nothing that he cannot do, but because of his cognitive problems, there is very little that he can do by himself.

From the team, we learned that Paul didn't know he was hungry. He could not eat because he didn't know he was hungry, but he would eat if prompted to do so. Paul is the most motivated individual you could ever meet, and since the brain injury he is just as keen to do the right thing, so when he was prompted, he did the right thing. He was very compliant and willing. The team helped me understand that he had problems with getting started, and with knowing when to stop again once he has started. I think if you talk about his issues, he could now talk to you about his brain injury and how it stops him from doing things but he can't apply it to the future. That is what makes it so hard for family.

Did you feel you could trust the professionals involved?

That meant trusting someone else to do my job: I wanted to, but it was a 'big deal'. It was the subtle things that I noticed, which did not seem to be obvious to the professionals. I needed them to acknowledge that they saw these problems too. They were little things like checking the doors and repeatedly counting the fish; it wasn't awful, but it wasn't usual behaviour. I wanted to trust them, but I was very nervous. While Paul was living with us, the team said they would look after him and said we should go on holiday. I had to look after the rest of my family too, but trusting them to look after Paul was incredibly hard. It turned out okay, and so we carried on. We rented the house at the end of the road for the independent living trial, so it was far enough away but close enough for us to help if needed. Just before Paul moved into his own place, I said to Richard 'You better guarantee this is safe.' I was trusting someone else to do my job. I wanted them to guarantee he would be okay. Anna helped me to let him go, and it worked out okay.

It was harder with non-specialist professionals because Paul comes across so well. I had needed to fight to make sure powerful agencies understood. Paul was subject to investigation about eligibility for benefits. Their forms are so generic, asking questions that Paul could answer simply. One that comes to mind was 'Can you wake up to an alarm clock?' Paul would respond 'Yes.' I needed to add the full detail, to avoid confusion (i.e. to answer 'Yes' but add 'As long as somebody prompts Paul every night to set the alarm clock'). What you have is a man who is really pleasant, really willing, really engaged, really motivated and really incapable. Social services and his birth mother decided Paul had capacity to manage his own care needs, and in doing so Paul decided that he did not need a support package. I had to apply to the Court of Protection to become his Welfare Deputy. The judge made very nice comments about the MDT and my family, which was heart-warming and puts your faith back in the system. You can trust them, once sure you've given them the information they need to understand Paul's needs (so they get it).

What was your experience of the medico-legal system?

The medico-legal system understands litigation risk, and capacity assessments. I was enraged when the lawyers told me the defendants had offered 90 per cent liability and had recommended that we accept; I wanted to fight. Who did they think they were insulting my son?! I had to accept the 90 per cent. I couldn't believe it. Lawyers need to be much more sensitive to a family's feelings, because they can be cheesed off, it was not his fault he got injured but he was blamed by 10 per cent.

The defendant's medical experts tell you when you walk in the door that they want to review your loved one's injury and will submit a report based on those findings. When you receive the reports, you wonder who they are talking about because it certainly wasn't my son on several of the appointments I took him on. I still, to this day, cannot understand how two highly qualified consultants cannot agree on the extent of a brain injury. The defendant's lawyers will send letters accusing your loved one of all sorts of different things, totally disagreeing with your lawyer's assessment of your loved one's disabilities. It's very unsettling.

To me, the law is not about right and wrong, it's about a load of old duffers, twisting and bending the rules, posturing and pushing to get into pole position, and this can go on for years. Your patience will be tried, you will be pushed and pulled in all directions wondering if it is all worth it, but it is the law. If you go to court again, to me it is not about the law, it is about who performs best.

After all this, most cases never go to court, they are settled between lawyers. I, along with Paul, went to our barrister's chambers in London. Two or three hours later we had a deal. The defendant's lawyers asked if they could see me, I agreed, remembering I wanted to physically fight them a few years before. I went in to the defendant's room; they told me Paul was lucky to have a father like me and wanted to meet me to tell me that they felt that I had only ever acted for Paul and had been nothing but fair.

That puts your faith back in the law.

Tell me about your feelings, your anger and how you coped in the early days.

I was angry when Paul got hurt, more than anything else because as his Dad I could not make him better or take the pain away. As a parent, I have one job – to protect my children, and when you can't, you feel so fragile, not a man, not the head of the family. You are a passenger on a train driven by others who know what's best for your child … but … hang on a minute … isn't that my job? Not anymore.

I sat in my bedroom and cried; my wife came in and I told her I just wanted to be in the coma rather than him; she said 'I know.' It's a bit of a coward's way out, but it was the fear of what I didn't know. I had a son who was asleep, I didn't know when he was going to wake up, who he would be or what he would be, I would rather be in his place because I didn't know how to deal with what was happening.

Once I accepted the reality of what had happened, I had to drop the work hard, play hard construction worker thing. I was a raw man, destroyed by an incident that lasted only a few seconds but would change our lives forever. I was a parent, reliant on my wife to counsel me. I had to have this outlet, someone who would listen, not judge, talk, not talk, comfort me. Anna quietly did this for me, all while coping with a baby, a toddler and a teenager. She is the strong one.

I am not angry with the NHS; at the point of need, Paul got the very best medical care. I was angry with people and organisations that I couldn't trust, who I didn't feel had Paul's welfare as their priority.

Tell me about Anna

I don't want to say that I am the one at the heart of this, for it is Paul who is at the heart of this story, yet Paul is the least aware of this story. So here I am, telling the story, but Anna has enabled me to do what I have done for Paul. She is under-recognised as part of it, for her commitment to Paul and me and this whole process has been selfless. Anna is the strong one; she is the one who continued on in spite of everything that is going on. She is the one that continued to look after the children when I sometimes sat and cried.

She quietly and patiently held the family together. She allowed me the time to focus on Paul, to spend as much time as I needed, or not, at the hospital. She was quietly picking up the pieces and making sure there was still a family there to go back to when I was ready to come back. Not until I look back after 17 years and talk to people who knew me at the time, do I realise how I probably wasn't functioning all that well in the weeks and months post-injury, even though I thought I was doing okay.

Anna was a constant prop for me. She and I worked as a team. I would have been screwed without her. She said 'Right … .your son has these problems … ' and she listed them, then she said 'We won't get anywhere by arguing with the care team. We need Richard so you need to find a way to work it out with him.' She could counsel me about what we needed as a family and she found a way to make me see why we need them and can't sack them all.

How have your feelings, and how you cope with them, shifted over the years?

It hurt then and it still hurts now. I tried shouting and it didn't work. That was what I did before.

I hate to think of him as damaged ... but you have to accept now where things are now ... that's what makes him and there is nothing I can do about it now, and I just have to accept how things are and crack on with it. That's what we do. I'm his dad and I'm obligated to be his dad until the day I die. I will not discharge my responsibility to another professional, but if they can help me then I am obligated to accept their help.

I owe him everything because I wasn't there to stop him from getting hurt that day. I hate it. This is not how it was supposed to be, but I haven't grieved for it, I don't know how. This is lifelong.

Although my son and I have a father–son relationship now, I can never see through the brain injury. When someone changes so much and you never properly grieve for the loss, it's natural that you cannot see through the injury. Its always there. I feel a conflict, a tension in me about what has happened and whether I ought to be thankful for what we have or grieve for what we have lost. In many ways, we have not lost anything because Paul has gone on to live a life with all the components in it that he might have had anyway ... he has a home, a wife, children, good relationships with his parents and his family. He doesn't miss what he didn't have. In contrast, the whole family know that something is different and that things could have been different. Am I being selfish to think of what I have lost, when he is not aware of what he has lost? Sometimes I feel like I need to grieve and I am full of sadness thinking about how this all is. I hate it. I hate what has happened. There are other people in the world who have worries and problems, and there is always somebody worse off than you, but I hate this situation. It is never-ending. Paul is at the best point we could have hoped for him, I love him and I'm proud of him and he's doing so much better than I imagined he would when I saw his head bleeding on 13th May 2001. But, he is not where he could have been. We will never know what could have been. We are struggling with this loss that doesn't really exist, and over the years we have struggled to get to know our son with a brain injury. That is what professionals are confronted with (or what is confronted in us, when we meet with professionals who tell us what they think we ought to be doing). That 'lost but not lost' thing, is the thing that is an obstacle, and which cannot be fixed.

Above all, he was not lucky (which is what everyone tells him – how lucky he was).

I wish this had never happened, but it has happened, and while I'm always aware of the loss I'm not always full of sadness and grief. Sometimes we laugh. Just because he has a brain injury now, it doesn't mean we can't laugh when he says or does something funny, and he is the same with us. Its not what we had planned, but this is our life now, this is our normal and this is how we live. This happened to our family, but we are still a happy, loving family.

What would you like to tell professionals?

Professionals who can get family 'buy in' at an early stage will get a much better outcome through the rehabilitation process. The family may resist, like me, but careful management of an over-protective father, taking a step back, not backing away or avoiding an awkward meeting, helped. Despite my initial belief that Paul could live with us, I was later convinced that Paul should attempt to live independently when the case manager came back with a care plan written by the whole team, including my wife. They listened, and they told me why they thought what they did, and I started to trust them. I would suggest to professionals that:

a   The initial meeting with the brain injured person should include the immediate family care givers. I think it would be good if they speak to the family members first, before trying to engage with their loved one. If they begin by talking about the loved one, and not about the family member's experience so far, family members will find it much harder to engage and get on board. Getting on board with the family, at least in our case, was crucial to getting Paul on board.

b   They need to remember that the family are new to this.

c   To me, and to other families perhaps, the first meeting feels threatening; I thought 'These people were going to encroach on my family. I have to do something.' Be sensitive. Go gently and listen.

What advice would you give to other families affected by brain injury?

Your child, partner, loved one is exactly that: yours. Set your aspirations high, never stop working for the best outcome; there will be a point at which you will realise that you are at a point when you are managing the outcomes of brain injury, and that will be fine: you may not have met your original aspiration but you got as close to it as you could.

Always remember you are acting in your loved one's 'best interests', which you will hear a lot. Best interests can also be called 'capacity', which is a legal term and can cover areas such as finance, welfare and care.

When you and your care team are working with your loved one, who is included, they are always working in his/her best interests, so this is a meeting with an agreed outcome between family and professionals. These MDT meetings can be overwhelming, but remember you know your loved one best, the team need your input to create an effective care package.

Capacity is something slightly different. If your loved one cannot manage their own affairs or work in their own best interests with the input of the MDT it may be necessary to question your loved one's capacity. This requires an application to the court of protection, which is easily done online and your MDT can help. An application to the court will be made on a single question, such as 'Can your loved one manage their own financial affairs?' It may be that you, with the MDT, advise your loved one to hold their money in the bank and make payments by direct debit. In reality, your loved one may draw all of their cash and spend it in the pub rather than paying bills – which s/he has every right to do, but would that person, with the advice, do that if they had not had a brain injury? If the answer is no an application to the court should be considered.

You should not be fazed by any of the above, you have gone through the most traumatic part of the process when your loved one acquired their brain injury. Everything you do from that point forward is focused on getting the best outcome; these are just tools to allow you to get to the point where your loved one can live an independent life, as close to your/their aspirational goals as possible.

On a different note, I want to say that in all of these bad bits, there are always little wins. There will be dark times but there will be little bits of light: for me, it was those things the lawyers said, and Anna. My wife smiling at me and saying its okay, you can cry, stare into space, shout, hit doors if you want (although you will have to redecorate later). My family and the care team put the little bits of light back into the darkness. There will always be something that enables you to get to the next day.

More recently, as I think about it, I have learned that it's okay to have changed too. This experience has changed me as a person. As a result of Paul's brain injury I have changed and improved in my communication skills and this has led to promotions at work. If I hadn't learned from it then perhaps I would have been too rigid, and the fact that I have learned from it shows that I have been flexible, and made changes, and so I have continued to do my best to help Paul to get to where he has got to.

What's important to you about writing this chapter?

Honesty.

There is no point in me telling this story if I am not honest.

What are you thankful for?

The last thing I said to our son on that Sunday morning before he went jet skiing with his friend was 'I love you.' Not for the sake of saying it, but because I did, that gives me comfort.

Summary and reflections

When Paul sustained a traumatic brain injury at the age of 15, his family were flung into a new reality. Dan tells the story of his family's journey through that terrible time. He described it as feeling out of control, like he was on a train that 'someone else was driving' and this meant other people telling him what was best for his son; something that sat uncomfortably with his personal values. The strength of his family loyalty and commitment to parenting prevented him from rejecting professionals and he was forced to find a way forward. Interestingly, Dan reflects on changes in himself over the years. He wonders whether the patience, confidence and communication skills he used in helping Paul have inadvertently helped his life elsewhere.

Engagement: does the team actually become part of the family?

When I asked Dan how it came to be that he was able to work with the team, to become part of the team, I was surprised that he turned it around and told me that to him it felt like the team had actually become part of his family. Of course! I had been looking at it through a professional's lens and of course, I had been blind to that point of view. Nonetheless, I thought this was an extraordinary turn around from the initial anger and rejection of the case manager who perhaps somehow represented the rude and abrupt intrusion of brain injury into this hard-working family's life. So, how does it happen that the enemy becomes the friend? It's essential, that in order to work together long term, the team must engage the family. Dan agreed. It's a process that happens in the first meeting, or maybe the first couple of meetings. Dan thinks it was possible because the professionals had the same interests, or we might say, the same 'values'. There is lots of literature which cites different points of focus to optimise the opportunities for building a working relationship (Oddy and Herbert, 2003, Sohlberg et al., 2001). For Dan, it was values associated with tattoos, camping and family, but for other people it will be different values of course. For Dan, it was important that working with him and Paul was a vocation and not just a job, that professionals explicitly recognised that family need does not diminish after 5 p.m. on a Friday.

Just as Dan learned from the professionals, we too are taught lessons by our clients. Some years ago now, I wrote about the importance of sharing power with families or the 'benign use of power' in building relationships with family members (Palmer, 2006, Bowen et al., 2010). In that project, the psychologist who sat on the floor in order to describe the formulation was described as helpful in engaging the family (i.e. making it safe to be honest). Dan similarly described the case manager sitting on the floor as a significant moment in their relationship; reducing the power differential and creating a safe space.

Grief, pride, commitment and attachment

Dan is on the brink of tears as he tells me, 17 years on, that his son is different. The depth of these emotions, held close for so long, is tangible and devastating. He stays with it for a while, his lip quivers and I know he is fighting with whether to be thankful or to allow himself a glimpse of the sadness that could engulf him, even now. He jumps up and gets a cuppa.

While he is away, I am thinking about attachment (Bartholomew, 1993) and the formation of safe relationships: 'Richard and I have probably learned from each other ... I think of him now as part of the family ... I have accepted him and others in the team and feel about them as if they were family'. I wonder what could have been his experience if he wasn't fortunate enough to find a case manager who contained his distress and became a secure attachment figure for him. I am thinking about the importance of how we manage power differentials in relationships to create space for the voice of the family to be properly heard.

Dan comes back with a smile and a change of conversation. I tell Dan my theory about attachment, and the significance of the patient yet persistent case manager in finding a way to connect with Dan. I share my theory that perhaps this is about professionals not only listening, but really hearing, and really respecting. He agrees: 'My aim is to provide the best I can for my family. The best I can. That means I must listen to the best people and accept that I may not always be the best one, and I cannot do it alone. Andy Murray may be doing all that fancy footwork but there is a whole massive team supporting him to get to that point. Richard helped me trust the team to help my boy.'

Thinking back to our first meeting …. As I sat, listening to Dan and Richard share reflections and jokes about the process, and refer to the intensity of feelings they both had, I am reminded of the importance not only of the parent's unswaying commitment to help his son, but also the case manager's unswaying commitment to engage with the parent; they are both tasked with the job of looking after the injured person. The respect on both sides is tangible. There is an honesty and openness that you can't bottle. I suppose it comes with time and a shared goal.

Family adjustment and coping

The literature about family adjustment post brain injury is too vast to summarise here (Blais and Boisvert, 2007, Bowen et al., 2009, Lezak, 1988, Perlesz et al., 1999) but this story highlights to me that, assuming the family intention is to act in the injured relative's best interests, it is absolutely crucial that professionals find a way of working alongside the values of the client and their family, in order to build the relationship and to include the family members in the planning and decision making, 'whatever it takes'. It is within that working relationship with the family system that the magic happens (Blow et al., 2007, Gaston, 1990, Horwitz et al., 1998). Family members are very often the most consistent persons that somebody has after brain injury, and finding ways of maximising their ability to understand and support their loved one is pivotal in functional outcome (Oddy and Herbert, 2003). As Dan knows, the family members are often best placed to then educate the professionals about subtle but significant ways in which their loved one needs support. Literature describes factors related to families *not* coping; the challenges that family members face as partners, parents and siblings (Gervasio and Kreutzer, 1997, Perlesz et al., 2000, Rivera et al., 2007). This story describes challenges consistent with previous research, but is much more about a family overcoming the adversity of brain injury, it is an uplifting, energising story about a family *coping*.

Although they did not immediately use it, the family found the information from Headway (Headway.org) helpful, which supports the current practice of continuing to give information and contact numbers in acute and post-acute care, which families can draw on when the time is right for them.

Dan tells the story of his family who have been through an enormous amount over the years (not only with the brain injury, but with other significant life events too) and they maintained a happy, loving family life. His straight-talking manner meant that he was able to put into words the worries and uncertainties of his family position during this long journey of recovery, rehabilitation and adjustment. Dan is animated, sensitive and honest in his description. Condensed into our coffee shop conversations, this story has been quite the rollercoaster for me too.

Patience, compassion and appreciating all the little things people do

I am reminded that there is a role for patience on both sides; the team allowing Dan to stand during meetings, and Dan to continue coming to meetings in spite of his discomfort. Arlene Vetere, one of my early mentors in systemic family therapy, taught me the importance of 'really getting to know the problem', to take time to understand the complexity of what was going on in the family, and avoiding the impulse to rush to a solution (Vetere and Dallos, 2003). Dan talks about Anna as under-recognised in this story. Anna represents patience in the face of complexity, and we are reminded of the importance of taking things slowly and being patient. I am reminded that there are many strands to family, and that the family continues to operate as a system in spite of the injury. The story reminds us of the juggling act that families are inevitably doing with the shopping, housework, childcare and their own emotions too (often behind the scenes) to just keep things going so they can come to the hospital to meet with the team. Recognising the roles of all the family members will add a richness and strength to your ultimate intervention. Literature on coping cites the benefits of task-oriented coping, but in the face of long-term problems (Collins et al., 1983) there is an important role for emotion-focussed coping. With the secure base of Anna and Richard, Dan was able to find his voice and shift away from task or avoidant coping, into a blend of task-and emotion-focussed coping strategies – an optimum position. It is these strategies that probably helped him find the patience and communication skills that enabled him to tell his story so eloquently today.

Although there is a strong argument for inclusion of family, it is sometimes very difficult to establish a shared understanding or shared goal between professionals and family members. Perhaps that it is where it is useful to draw on pre-injury information about family relationships and narratives. Family adjustment is a process, and Dan describes his experience over the last 17 years. The narrative may have been different if we had spoken at different time points.

Is there a happy ending?

After everything I've heard, I dare to ask Dan if there is a happy ending; 'Certainly', he boldly says '... this is a story of being a family "no matter what". There will always be sad things, but these awful times also teach us about ourselves. With the support of each other, we have got so much further than we thought we could, and we are closer and tighter as a family than ever before.' He went on to tell me: 'I've been through this process, and it's changed me. I'll never be able to properly explain how I feel about it, but I've met a wonderful OT, two wonderful neuropsychologists, and Paul has two kids so I also have wonderful grandchildren. He has a wife who makes him happy and I have a friend for life in the case manager; I have a really happy life. If that's not a happy ending, I don't know what is!'

Speaking to other families, he says 'As a family, we have all put a huge part of our own lives into supporting Paul to help him achieve his ambition to be the best dad that he can, and I think he has achieved it. I want other families to know that it will get better, and there will be a happy ending. You don't think so, but those little bits of light will become brighter. I never thought they would, but we have found them as a family and my family are those bits of light for me. We know that every time we walk out of the door it might be the last time. We live with grief. We did not allow our family to fall apart, and we took the professionals into our family which made us all stronger. Like scaffolding, but I don't know who scaffolds who.'

I felt nervous when we shook hands at the end of our meeting. The fragility of life is right up at the front of my mind as we shake hands. 'I hope you have a safe journey home .... thank you for everything' ... and there we go, on our different journeys. This story resonates with me. It reminds me that every story needs to be heard. The more we listen, the more responsive, creative and broadminded we can be as clinicians, which in turn means we give ourselves better skills to work with families and help more individuals see the glints of light.

References

Bartholomew, K. 1993. From childhood to adult relationships: attachment theory and research. In: *Learning about relationships* (Duck, S., ed.). Understanding Relationship Processes series, vol. 2. Thousand Oaks, CA: Sage.

Blais, M.C., & Boisvert, J.M. 2007. Psychological adjustment and marital satisfaction following head injury: which critical personal characteristics should both partners develop? *Brain Injury*, 21, 357–372.

Blow, A.J., Sprenkle, D.H., & Davis, S.D. 2007. Is who delivers the treatment more important than the treatment itself? The role of the therapist in common factors. *Journal of Marital Family Therapy*, 33, 298–317.

Bowen, C., Hall, T., Newby, G., Walsh, B., Weatherhead, S., & Yeates, G. 2009. The impact of brain injury on relationships across the lifespan and across school, family and work contexts. *Human Systems: The Journal of Consultation and Training*, 20, 65–80.

Bowen, C., Yeates, G., & Palmer, S.O.N. 2010. *A relational approach to rehabilitation: thinking about relationships after brain injury*. London: Karnac.

Collins, D.L., Baum, A., & Singer, J.E. 1983. Coping with chronic stress at Three Mile Island: psychological and biochemical evidence. *Journal of Health Psychology*, 2, 149.

Gaston, L. 1990. The concept of the alliance and its role in psychotherapy: theoretical and empirical considerations. *Psychotherapy: Theory, Research, Practice, Training*, 27, 143.

Gervasio, A.H., & Kreutzer, J.S. 1997. Kinship and family members' psychological distress after traumatic brain injury: a large sample study. *Journal of Head Trauma Rehabilitation*, 12, 14–26.

Horwitz, R.C., Horwitz, S.H., Orsini, J., Antoine, R.L., & Hill, D.M. 1998. Including families in collaborative care: impact on recovery. *Journal of Families, Systems and Health*, 16, 71.

Lezak, M.D. 1988. Brain damage is a family affair. *Journal of Clinical and Experimental Neuropsychology: Official Journal of the International Neuropsychological Society*, 10, 111–123.

Oddy, M., & Herbert, C. 2003. Intervention with families following brain injury: evidence-based practice. *Neuropsychological Rehabilitation*, 13, 259–273.

Palmer, S. 2006. Understanding and coping: family members' experience of rehabilitation services. *Brain Impairment*, 7, 162.

Perlesz, A., Kinsella, G., & Crowe, S. 1999. Impact of traumatic brain injury on the family: a critical review. *Rehabilitation Psychology*, 44, 6–35.

Perlesz, A., Kinsella, G., & Crowe, S. 2000. Psychological distress and family satisfaction following traumatic brain injury: injured individuals and their primary, secondary, and tertiary carers. *Journal of Head Trauma Rehabilitation*, 15, 909–929.

Rivera, P., Elliott, T.R., Berry, J.W., Grant, J.S., & Oswald, K. 2007. Predictors of caregiver depression among community-residing families living with traumatic brain injury. *NeuroRehabilitation*, 22, 3–8.

Sohlberg, M.M., McLaughlin, K.A., Todis, B., Larsen, J., & Glang, A.J. 2001. What does it take to collaborate with families affected by brain injury? A preliminary model. *Journal of Head Trauma Rehabilitation*, 16, 498–511.

Vetere, A., & Dallos, R. 2003. *Working systemically with families: formulation, intervention and evaluation*. London and New York: Karnac.

Chapter 4

Behaviour, vulnerability and the criminal justice system

This chapter is a collaboration between a mother, Jeanne, and Jackie Dean (Occupational Therapist and Brain Injury Case Manager). Following a lengthy telephone conversation, it was agreed that Jeanne would start by putting her story in writing. This took some time and subsequent emails noted that this had involved the whole family and had been a highly emotional experience. I was overtly aware that this was an extremely important piece of narrative and that it carried great emotional investment. I was reminded that professionals should remember the power of narrative in the healing process, and the importance of listening well.

Jeanne's story

My story is about the experience and struggles we went through as a family and all the obstacles we had to overcome to deal with brain injury and come to terms with the losses involved. I hope others can learn from our experience.

From boy to man

We moved to the south of England for Roger's job when Adam was 13.

As a child Adam was diagnosed as 'hyperactive', ADHD in today's language, which made him extremely energetic; he always needed to exhaust his physical energy before he was ready to learn. He was an intelligent, quick learner and excellent at any sport he chose to undertake, especially football, swimming, and running – he was always last baton in the relay races as he could save the day with his speed. In his first year at secondary school he was the school chess champion, winning trophies for his school; he was always a much sought-after footballer. Adam was very popular, a leader, never a follower, he had very many friends who he took care of, often bringing home 'stray lambs' asking could they stay, I always squared it with their parents. He had a great sense of humour, could always make us laugh with a funny story of 'guess what happened to me today'. He was wilful and would battle for his own way. He had a younger sister and all his five cousins were girls who adored him so he learned very early how to be with girls, which made girls very attracted to him in his teenage years, which in turn made him popular with his peers. He had the ability to pass exams without doing much revision, and passed his driving test first time at 17. He liked being independent, doing his own cooking and washing from an early age. He grew up very much as an individual full of charm and energy ready to make his way in the world. He was described as being 'A Cool Dude with attitude'. He took a job in an estate agents which was also a bank and building society. At the time of his accident at the age of 20 he was in training to become a manager. They had spotted a bright young man with potential. He was all grown up.

The accident (Adam's 21st birthday)

'Mum dad get up Adam has had a car accident JUST GET UP!' our daughter Anne was screaming at 3 a.m. A number of young people had gone out to celebrate Adam's 21st birthday and came back to our house to continue partying. Anne was in the house making food when the accident happened. We all ran down our garden to the road to find an upturned car. The boy who had been in the back was shouting over and over 'I couldn't get out of the car, I couldn't get out of the car', he was OK but limping, Anne took hold of him. My son was stretched out on his back in the road, one of the girls was a trainee nurse, she had hold of his wrist, she was shouting, 'I can't get a pulse.' I remember screaming and someone pushed another boy towards me, his forehead was flapping and he was covered in blood, he collapsed in my arms and I wrapped my cardigan around his bleeding head. Another young man was on his phone, 'RTA where the hell is the ambulance?' The police arrived but didn't help and just wanted to know who was driving. Eventually three ambulances arrived, there seemed to be flashing lights everywhere, and the paramedics started to work on my son straight away. I heard one say, 'OK he's breathing.'

Roger, Anne and another boy went with the boys in the ambulances. I ran back to the house to check on my 8-year-old son, he was still sleeping. I rang the parents of the other two boys to tell them to go to the hospital, then I rang my best friend who lived next door, 'Adam has had a car accident and I need you.' She came straight away to find me standing in my blood-stained nightie shaking in my bedroom. She dressed me and said, 'Come on, we have to get to the hospital.'

The other parents started to arrive, we all waited and waited. Finally they came to say the other two boys would be OK, one needed to be admitted for surgery on his head wound but our son was being sent to intensive care as he had a major brain injury and they had sent for the neurosurgeon.

Early next morning, Adam's girlfriend Amy, who hadn't been there the night of the accident, Roger, Anne and I sat at Adam's bedside bewildered by all the machinery and bleeping noises when the surgeon arrived. He had looked at the MRI and came with his diagnosis. 'So sorry your son has a major brain injury to his left temporal lobe, a fractured skull and a massive bleed, his brain is swelling, and we anticipate it will swell to such proportion it will press on his brain stem and we have no way of stopping it, it's just a matter of time. I am afraid I can't give you much hope other than a miracle.'

We knew the machines were keeping him alive, Adam was a fighter, but this could not help him now. The hospital pastor came to pray with me, he came to help me let my son go and I wasn't ready for that. By the third day our son was being prayed for all over the world, our village had a church service for him, the church was overflowing with well-wishers, prayers were all we had for hope. Then they came and mentioned tests to decide whether to turn the machines off, I said 'NO!', Roger said, 'You're not listening to them,' the neurosurgeon said, 'OK one more scan.' The surgeon came into the waiting room with the results, he was almost skipping: 'His brain has suddenly stopped swelling, I can't explain it other than we have our miracle.' After that hospital staff called Adam 'The Miracle Boy.'

The recovery

Amy, Adam's partner of two years who had been living with us, was given a bed some nights at the hospital to be on hand. Adam couldn't breathe on his own, so they gave him a tracheostomy and stopped all of the medication to bring him round from the induced coma he was in; this was hard to watch as he was shaking with drug withdrawals and his skin was all red and pimpled (cold turkey). They said he wouldn't remember. When he came round he was in a vegetative state; slavering, couldn't hold his head up, paralysed down one side, no speech and no control of his eyes or any of his bodily functions. He was unable to communicate and didn't recognise anyone; we were told to not expect much more due to the enormity of his injuries.

They needed the bed in ITU so sent him on to a general ward; the first night he fell out of his bed. The next day we organised a daily rota with Amy, Anne and us so someone was there all the time. Roger slept with him on a mattress on the floor overnight because they did not have the staff to cope, our input was welcomed. We went to his therapies with him; they were not consistent so we started to do the therapies with him daily. He kept pulling his feeding tube out and I begged them to let me try to feed him; they gave me 24 hours then the tube would go back in. I achieved it spoon-feeding him, the tube did not go back in.

As soon as Adam could stand Roger and I got him between our shoulders and taught him to put one foot in front of the other; he started fighting back and his physical progress was remarkable. Each night when I got home, I would put a message on the answer machine about his progress to update all callers. They left messages of support which was wonderful to listen to after a hard day at the hospital. Casseroles and the like kept appearing on the doorstep, we had no family close so all this was most welcome. Eventually my aunt and uncle came to stay for six weeks to run the household, so we could spend the time with Adam. We had a 24 hour rota of family and friends for constant attendance and kept a book logging his daily progress. He learned to walk, be in control of his bodily functions and talk albeit he seldom made any sense. He had regressed into being a very young child, very frightened and unable to make sense of the world. He was verbally and sometimes physically aggressive, his way of fighting back in a world he didn't understand any more. A child in a man's body, a psychological state that he still presents with now which has been the most difficult personality change to manage.

A month after his accident Adam's best friend George, also aged 21, who had been visiting Adam every day, came off his push bike and a metal railing spike pierced his head. We were at his bedside with his parents and sister when they turned the machines off, we attended the funeral. Roger read a tribute to George who had been a constant member of our household spending holidays and the previous Christmas with us. We were unable to tell Adam of George's death for some time, we told him he was with relatives on holiday. I remember feeling guilty for fighting so hard to keep my son alive when George's mother lost hers; it almost felt like an unfair price to be paid. Further down the line I worked through George's death and my guilt feelings in counselling, I needed this as this was the thing that kept me strong enough to cope. Through counselling I was able to acknowledge the trauma of being at the scene and work through the ongoing grieving process that comes with the loss of who the person was before. Because I got this help, I was able to support my family, albeit the grief is ever present for us all as we are confronted daily through our struggles with what is and what has gone from our lives. The son we have today is not the son I gave birth to and nurtured into a man. When times got tough I would tell Adam he had to live two lives now, one for him and one for George. When he was able he would go and sit next to George's grave and talk to him, he never stopped missing his best friend. George's parents split up after his death.

Rehabilitation

Finally Adam was sent to a Brain Injury Rehabilitation Unit. I went every weekday after I collected our youngest son Robbie from school, a 100-mile round trip. Anne went Mondays and Roger, Robbie and I went weekends as well as Adam's friends. Adam discovered how to ring me from a payphone with reverse charges and rang me at least 15 times daily asking me to go and get him. He thought they were trying to harm him and was afraid most of the time. He would only have a bath when I arrived as he thought they would try to drown him and he would only settle to sleep after I had tucked him up in his bed. Often he had put all his belongings in a suitcase and he and his case could be found in various hiding places behind curtains etc. This was all part of his regressive state. He wanted me to bring him sweets, something he had not been a fan of throughout his life before. Amy his girlfriend, supported by her mother, left him; she decided she was unable to cope with the post-injury Adam, but he kept asking for her. I remember feeling angry and let down at the time. Now I do understand.

The neuropsychologist in charge at the rehabilitation unit called me in. He came to the conclusion Adam would be better living at home and travelling in initially daily then reducing to one day per week and then after a short period to none. He thought Adam would realise his cognitive impairments better through struggling in the community, as Adam was oblivious to any of his limitations within the protected environment of the rehabilitation centre. Adam was released into my care.

Overcoming brain injury and the struggles

I remember people saying 'Hasn't he been lucky?' and 'Aren't you lucky?' because he came back to us looking 'normal' on the outside. My sister was angry because as she put it, 'We never see you now because you are so wrapped up in Adam.' Roger's family hadn't come to visit Adam and had no idea of what we were coping with. It was something that was hard to put into words when we didn't understand it ourselves.

Roger was back at work and I was left to take charge of Adam without any education or instruction, not knowing what to expect. I asked for a visit from a social worker. When she arrived, Adam was still in bed late morning; she said 'Oh I have a lazy teenager just like him, I see your profession is a psychotherapist, well you are the best person to care for him, we barely have enough funding for our elderly.' Then she finished her tea, said goodbye and left without even seeing him. I knew nothing about benefits and it was to be the following year before I discovered I could claim anything.

I learned about the deficits post brain injury on the hoof through experiencing his: memory loss, anger outbursts, mood swings, disinhibited behaviour issues, cognitive understanding and processing problems, loss of all executive functioning ability, lack of insight and personality change. I had to become: Mother, Nurse, Teacher and Carer to deal with my son. I was on duty day and night amid the trauma all the family was going through.

At the time his brother Robbie was only 8 years old and his sister Anne was 17. Robbie had not been allowed to visit in intensive care and until his aunt and uncle came to stay and help he had been farmed out to friends. He had concluded his brother was dead and we were not telling him; he started to overeat, which I failed to notice. He's now aged 30, has had driving lessons but been unable to drive; when I asked him why he said, 'Mum I don't want the responsibility.' He deals with Adam the best of all of us because he says he doesn't have much recollection of how he was before, therefore accepts him as he is.

Anne had been at the scene of the accident and seen her beloved brother fighting for his life on life support being fed through tubes; she felt guilty for eating when he couldn't and leaving him at night to go and get food; she stopped eating, which I failed to notice until one day I saw her thin little body coming up the drive. Her habit of not eating by then was an established pattern and became an on-going struggle for her. Today at age 40 she struggles with a condition called lupus which I believe could be as a result of the whole trauma.

The dynamics of the whole family changed. Adam, the big strong independent older brother, became the youngest and most dependent and the whole household revolved around him and his needs. Roger found respite in his heavy workload, coming home to be confronted with angry unacceptable behaviour he didn't understand from Adam.

Roger was also trying to take care of me, seeing me being stretched and stressed with two other children always waiting in the wings, putting their needs on the back burner. Adam was the big baby cuckoo in our nest.

Adam's behaviour was problematic, he had unpredictable anger outbursts where he would punch holes in the wall and I would cover over with yet another picture. He would punch out and I would get under this 6'3" man and hold him around his waist and say, 'You're OK I'm here.' He never hurt me. I realized he was not able to cry, and all his emotions were expressed through anger. His language was inappropriate, and Robbie's friends were not allowed to come to our house because of his older brother's aggressive behaviour and foul language, nor was he invited back to theirs any more. Adam wanted to play with them, which appeared weird to their mothers. Robbie was getting bullied at school because his brother was odd; he was sad, not sociable anymore and fat. His best friend since they were aged 2 told him his mother had told him not to be friends with Robbie any more, Robbie just kept eating. Anne's female friends hated coming to the house as Adam was inappropriate and suggestive to them. This lack of boundaries was to be a major issue. Adam's friends had dropped off as instead of him being the leader he was, he needed looking after and I guess they felt he held them back. They attempted to take him on holiday to Tenerife and I had to send Anne out there to bring him back from hospital where he was recovering from a series of seizures due to being left to go off with the wrong company where they fed him drugs and booze.

Adam was unable to hold conversations or form any opinions. He was and still is easily led by others, he fits in with what is being said giving the impression he is engaging which for short periods can seem convincing. He doesn't have a stop button, easily gets overloaded and can flip into an angry response very quickly. When with people who were unable to manage him, he got into trouble. His lack of insight and inability to censor what he said would also lead him into trouble. Anne and his father tried to be with him when he insisted on going to the local pub. Adam had a sense of feeling he was invincible. Anne often found herself defending him, saying, 'He's got a brain injury, he can't help it.' Stopping him was not always possible. Unfortunately, that wilfulness from childhood became exaggerated and he was very much a child wanting his own way in a man's physically strong body. He used his aggression as power as this was all the power he had. When he couldn't win an argument with his younger brother, he would hit him, so I was not able to leave them alone.

After 2 years somehow, Anne completed her A levels and got a place at university. She deferred and went travelling with a friend then she came home for a summer and left for uni. We moved house from our little village to a town to enable Adam to be more independent. Robbie changed schools. Solutions? Not really, just different beginnings.

I started working again, part time, evenings and weekends. An old girlfriend of Adam's who he had been very fond of in his teens had been spending time with him, she had lots of problems of her own and she moved in with us. They struck up a relationship and within 2 years post-injury she was pregnant. She thought, like us, that it was just a matter of time before Adam would gain his old self back, he was with her throughout the pregnancy and we celebrated the birth of our first girl grandchild. As soon as the baby was born, she left him and went to live at her mother's. We visited her and the baby there. Adam couldn't understand why she didn't want him anymore. This was to be a long on-off relationship as Adam was obsessed with her as he had been as a teenager.

Anne graduated and in her final year met an Australian boyfriend. She went to live with him in Australia. Anne didn't really address the 'loss' of her brother until years later, I think she just pushed on with her life in denial; to me it felt like she needed to run away; it brought more loss and sadness into our lives albeit we were happy for her. We wanted to hate her new boyfriend, but he is so lovely we learned to love him and his family. They got married and continue to live in Australia very happily with their two lovely boys. I started childminding Adam's child which helped us cope with Anne leaving.

Adam regained his love of cars and started driving again after being tested and given the OK. He wanted to work again to have some money, he could see his friends earning and getting on and he was jealous of their success. Roger took him to work with him, gave him a few little office jobs to do and tried to introduce him to working again. Even with his Dad's support Adam was unable to be reliable and maintain concentration long enough. So, we tried him with physical work, washing cars as he loved cars; again he was unable to work independently or maintain any regular attendance. He was easily distracted and lacked motivation and any feeling of responsibility or commitment.

We took him to a careers officer, who couldn't suggest much by way of training. We asked Social Services to come back and assess him. They said they could only help him if we threw him out, then they could pick up the case especially if he was homeless! Again the 'lazy' word came up with them as they left. This time I did make a complaint, to be told they were not trained in brain injury.

Adam started going out with wild males much younger than himself and he became promiscuous, not using contraception. I guess his mental age was about 14. He was a target for those who took advantage of vulnerable people and he kept company with females who usually came from dysfunctional backgrounds. He almost had to prove he was still a man by drinking too much, which got him into trouble.

The mother of his child moved back into the area and they slowly became friends again, he moved in with her and before long she was pregnant again. She gave birth to another beautiful girl and shortly afterwards threw him out. She was unable to cope with his immaturity. He was devastated and found solace in alcohol. We had access to both children mainly as childminders.

My father came to live with us, he was diagnosed with vascular dementia and the family sent him to me to care for. I got Adult Social Care involved for him and they were very helpful in getting him referred to two dementia day centres. Adam was brilliant with him, they 'got' each other. Dad got worse very quickly. I was up at nights again, and it became too much for me. It was Dad or Adam, I couldn't get Adam housed anywhere else as he had a history of aggression, and by now he had two convictions for drunk driving and ABH. Roger and I re-mortgaged our house and purchased a house around the corner for Adam, he moved in with a longstanding friend of his who promised to be a good carer. Up to a point it worked as Adam came around to me every day, but I was unable to monitor his night time activities of mainly getting drunk and mixing with the wrong sort of people; unfortunately his friend was also a drinker.

We had the children every Saturday, his ex would drop them at Adam's house and I would go round, they would argue in front of the children and eventually he struck her and she fell over. She went to the police and he was arrested. Yet again, as the responsible adult in his life, I found myself at the police station. This time we both got locked in a holding cell for 10 hours until they decided to interview him. The solicitor advised us not to mention the brain injury as it would be detrimental rather than do any good. He was convicted with a suspended sentence and tagged for three months, being confined to his house nightly for 12 hours. His friend left as they too had been fighting. Adam came to us in the day and I had to keep him company many nights; he became depressed; I found out later he was drinking through the nights. One night when I was unable to be there, he rang me to say he had cut the tag off and was going to throw himself under a train. I managed to find him; the tag cutting had been reported. We went back to court and requested he be released from the tag as due to the brain injury he was unable to tolerate being tagged. The magistrate put up her hand and said 'we will not be subjected to these feeble excuses, a crime has been proven and the punishment stands'. The request was refused and because he was suicidal, I sought help from the mental health team where he was allocated a Community Psychiatric Nurse. They referred him to Headway for 6 weeks rehabilitation, which was funded; this was 10 years post-injury. Hope at last.

My father died and Adam took up with a girl who turned out to have problems with her immigration status; she moved in with him. Their relationship was not easy, they had fights, and whilst in this relationship he got into a fight where he was outnumbered and badly beaten. He ended up in hospital having to have reconstruction surgery to his face, again all fuelled by alcohol consumption. She eventually left his/our house at my request. Adam became depressed and was afraid to go out for fear of being attacked again. Through our doctor I requested he see a neuropsychologist. We waited nine months for the appointment; in the meantime I had supported him through this without any outside support.

Adam attended a furniture restoration project for people with mental health difficulties. He enjoyed it and learned a lot of paint techniques. Unfortunately, he met an older woman there with significant mental health issues and they had a relationship which ended badly in a physical fight; this time they had both been smoking drugs and drinking. The police were called and Adam was arrested. He was facing another ABH court case, which being a fourth offence would carry for sure a custodial sentence.

At that time, I was working for Headway as a Group Facilitator with brain injured clients and their carers. I had had a lot of education and training on the subject of brain injury. From my past experience of the law's negative, uneducated attitude and lack of knowledge of the needs of brain injured offenders, I decided to put up a fight to keep my son from going to prison. I spent a whole summer researching the law, educating the solicitor on brain injury symptoms and gathering evidence of his post-brain injury deficits. I got him assessed by a neuropsychologist who did a report alongside Headway's assessment from his time with them; I got in contact with everyone in the brain injury field who had had any dealings with Adam to write about him. As expected, he was convicted but the sentence needed to be appropriate. I had a meeting with his probation officer and she asked for the court psychologist to access him and also submit a report. I got him accepted into a live-in assessment and rehab programme at a specialist centre in London, which funding was never granted for, and he started attending Alcohol Education and Counselling. The court psychologist said, if he got a custodial sentence, she would get him out under a specific section of the Mental Health Act.

To our relief he got a fine and a 12-month suspended sentence; the court listened to the argument put forward and I believe psychological assessments have been regularly used by that court since then. What a breakthrough.

Conclusion

Life doesn't take you on the journey you want; with brain injury there is not enough understanding or information about all the issues involved for the brain injured person and their families. Cuts in funding make us a fire-fighting society; once the hospital fight is over and survival is achieved, that is the NHS' job done. The real fight begins when battling for the best recovery possible for the injured person and their family. This is where I, my family and many others have been let down. I think if our family had been given information about what happens after brain injury and support to deal with outcomes from the outset, we may have coped better.

Currently I am volunteering as part of a team set up by Headway East Sussex, offering a Hospital Liaison Service which is being welcomed by hospital staff who are already stretched with their nursing duties. We go into hospitals to; give out information leaflets, offer advice, support and direction to all services, to help brain injured patients and their families, consider what they may need after discharge from hospital. It is well documented that early rehabilitation is more beneficial, as is supporting and educating families. This Headway Hospital Liaison Service is headed up by a paid member of Headway staff. Headway receives no state funding whatsoever for this. Paid Headway staff run an ongoing follow-up service to check if patients/carers are coping further down the line.

Headway applied for lottery money to help run this service with the intention of including more hospitals. It was refused on the grounds that this service is already in force through NHS. In our view and our experience, it is not.

For me, education was the key to helping me when I was struggling in the dark. Learning through my difficult experiences without support made the journey harder. Once I learnt, I was able to educate others, in particular our granddaughters, and enable them to understand why a Dad they love so much is so embarrassing.

Loss and grief also needs to be addressed. Our Headway runs a free counselling service for those on low income. The loss faced for all concerned is the hardest form of grief, the loss of what was when we still have them with us, is the most difficult grieving process to go through. They are here, but it's not them, we grab onto glimpses of what was, hoping they will come back. We feel sadness for them, sadness for us, whilst people say:

'Aren't you/they LUCKY.'

There is much more to Adam's story and many more incidents; these are just ones in the forefront of my mind. Today 23 years on he lives in another town with his wife of three years and her three teenage children. He is the main carer to their two small children: a boy aged 4 and baby girl aged 12 months. His eldest girl who lives with us is to be 21 this year and his other girl who lives with her mother will be 16. It's a hard life for him on many levels; he struggles on low income and still has problems within personal relationships. He has no social life and doesn't see any of his friends any more. He and his children visit us every Sunday and we do what we can to help. He's safe, he's loved and we talk about why he survived. To become a dad of course, as his four children are his life and his absolute pride and joy.

They are as precious to him as he has always been to us.

Professional perceptions

Jackie Dean, Occupational Therapist and Case Manager, has been working in the field of brain injury for many years, and reflects and responds to Jeanne's narrative.

Jeanne begins her account stating that her story is '*about the experience and struggles we went through as a family and all the obstacles we had to overcome to deal with brain injury and come to terms with the losses involved*'. I was struck in my conversation with her on the phone, as her written account unfurled, and by the email that accompanied her story when it arrived on my desk, to note that still '*many tears have been shed*' during the preparation and reading of her story, and that the family, whilst having made adjustments, continue to miss '*their precious son*'. I was struck by the vividness and detail of her account of the accident. A life-changing moment which continues to haunt her days.

This family were desperately clinging to hope or 'a miracle' during these first few weeks. I was struck by Jeanne's account of fighting with the team in the Intensive Care Unit for 'one more chance' and her strong drive to maintain control. They consider they were blessed as, against the odds, Adam survived. He is reported as being called 'miracle boy'.

As to be expected, Jeanne's focus had to remain on Adam at the inevitable expense of normal life, usual responsibilities were deferred and other family members were left with unmet needs. I noticed Jeanne wrote about the impact on Adam's siblings, and her own associated guilt. Jeanne describes her other children as damaged but having moved on. She detailed Robbie's difficulties and described those of Adam's sister, who took many years to accept help for the eating disorder that evolved following the accident, as a consequence of her unresolved guilt. She is described as pushing on with her life 'in denial' and seemed to 'want to run away'.

Adam did not have access to a significant amount of neuro-rehabilitation as an in-patient, as he had difficulty engaging as a consequence of his fear, confusion and impaired insight. He was discharged home on the basis that he lacked insight into his difficulties and needed to go home to experience problems. I was struck that this was a family that were being set up to fail without adequate support and resources. Sadly, in my experience this is not uncommon and there remains a paucity of specialist community services.

Adam did not have any community support other than his family. The expectations of community living were too demanding for him, and there is no doubt that specialist rehabilitation support would have proved invaluable, if provided at the right time.

I experience on a regular basis that assessments will refer to the person's cognitive and physical needs in detail but merely define that there are 'personality changes' or that the person is disinhibited without adequate analysis and consideration. Jeanne describes her son as the 'cuckoo in the nest' and that the 'son we have today is not the son that I gave birth to and nurtured into a man'.

It is important that professionals begin to place increasing emphasis on the wider family and have more understanding that the brain injury does not occur to the person in isolation, but in a real world. We need to focus on the context of that person within a family. Families cope best by having long term support. In order to have resilience they must learn how to adapt to the new life and make sure they take care of their health and wellbeing into the longer term.

Professionals do not always fully appreciate the challenges faced by family members. Expectations of family may be high, and lack of professional knowledge and impaired communication can lead to misinterpretations and families become labelled as 'over-involved', taking over, or inappropriate. Family members often become disregarded.

Empathy can be difficult for professionals to give, particularly where the professional has no understanding of brain injury, as in the 'non'-assessment by the social worker in this case, or where the support system around the person is under pressure, is disintegrating and is continuing to 'fight' and express anger, bewilderment and mistrust of the system. In this situation Jeanne discovered her former coping strategies were no longer helpful; she became immobilised, stuck and exhausted.

At the formative age when Adam, and many young people sustain their injuries, they are discovering themselves and developing independence. Identity is mixed up within a social context. Adam is described as a leader, sportsman, intelligent and independent prior to his accident, and afterwards negatively associated with his impulsive behaviours and presenting challenges. Adam lacks insight initially and over time, after negative experiences his self-identity changes and he develops 'depression'.

Adam's family, his friends and Adam himself had a certain perception of who Adam was. The accident not only places a grenade in the family, but there is a 'ticking time bomb' associated with not helping the injured person to identify a new role, and find the new person they have become, alongside assisting family and friends to also adjust. Jeanne comments that Adam's youngest brother, who had less memory and expectation of his brother before the accident, has accommodated him best. He is, however, impacted by the loss of his family structure and relationships

Adam was 21 when his accident occurred. This is a formative period and a time when the frontal systems of the brain are still undergoing maturation. The person is adjusting to community living, adulthood, and complex social interactions. As a result of the brain injury, Adam has difficulty in formulating goals, planning and problem solving, and effectively carrying out his plans, meaning that he responds impulsively or reactively to the environment without regard for the consequences. Inability to generate or initiate a plan, and resultant inactivity or a habitual response, despite advice, is often misunderstood as 'lazy', as in Adam's case, or as emotionally disturbed or malingering.

Adam is described as 'childish', 'insensitive' and 'aggressive'. He is reported to have had difficulty modifying his emotions, leading to repeated socially inappropriate behaviours, for example drinking to excess, becoming grossly indiscriminate in his approach to sexual partners, and being arrested for drink driving and assault. His changes in behaviour and poor social awareness has resulted in increasing social isolation from his peers and ultimately family members. Jeanne describes this disintegration powerfully. The inability to delay (or inhibit) action when aroused often contributes to poor choices, which in turn for Adam led to devastating social consequences.

This formative age of 21 is a time when people often present to services or to the criminal justice system with significant behavioural challenges, as they become involved in increasingly complex social situations. The impact of the brain injury on an ability to monitor behaviour, to self-regulate and correct mistakes causes ongoing and repeated 'disinhibited' behaviours. This is particularly the case where insight and self-awareness is impaired, and/or there is difficulty in identifying social cues.

In Adam's case this led to aggressive behaviour and certainly left him vulnerable to maleficent others. These difficulties after brain injury often lead to increasing social isolation, and the associated vulnerability can lead to seeking the company of people who will readily accept their 'odd behaviours'. Combined with difficulties with planning and memory, Adam has also had difficulty maintaining appointments and seeking out services, and conclusions were drawn by the social worker that he was unwilling to engage and did not need rehabilitation services or support, when this was far from the truth. Regrettably these conclusions were drawn despite consistent and clear evidence from family and others that Adam was not able to function in the real world, was at risk and in need of services.

The importance of a therapeutic alliance with an experienced practitioner cannot be underestimated. In essence, it does not matter how skilled a professional you are, in practice you also need to be able to communicate with the person in a meaningful way. Adam and his family have not had the opportunity to develop a relationship with a professional experienced in brain injury. It is saddening that he was at the point of a jail sentence when he found a professional that was able to support Jeanne to advocate on her son's behalf. The quality of the therapeutic relationship is critical in developing a meaningful rehabilitation programme and demands a skilled professional. Partnership is key, along with placing the person at the centre of the process, rather than a rigid adherence to processes that result in disjointed rehabilitation and services that do not fit need. Brain injury rehabilitation and support must be bespoke to the individual.

When reading Jeanne's account of Adam and her family's story, I am reminded of the fact, often easy to forget, that one instant on a single day is all that separates my life from those of the people that I work with. Each story, each life is unique, but in common there is a rippling of a tsunami of impacts across a person, their family, friends and community. Every day I am humbled by the tenacity and resilience of those I am privileged to meet.

The following poem was written by Anne not long after her brother Adam's brain injury:

Poem for My Big Brother

Always together but not always close,
Love's always there in some sort of dose.
Yet as years went by our love matured,
And together hard times were endured.

As family we've been like cat and mouse,
Shared the same bed or rooms in the house.
The jokes I've withstood and bruises I've worn
Have all been through love in some shape or form.

The jealousy and hate you felt for me,
Has faded with time and left us just free
To love one another and uncover our bond
Of brother and sister of which I am fond.

As children you became like a god,
For me to admire and withstand every prod.
And now though hurting I know you'll recover,
As I know I'm not going to lose my big brother.

I feel your pain, your hurt and frustration,
And my heart goes out in sheer desperation,
To heal your wounds and make things alright,
To help spread your wings and lift you to flight.

For this I'll wait till you're better in health
And you've had some time to do it yourself.
Then I'll be here with a helping hand,
To support you and love you and help you to stand.

As to recover I am sure you will manage,
And come through with the slightest of damage.
Cos you have to as I know you'll never bend
As life without you I can't comprehend.

So with all my heart I'm here for you,
To support you when you need me to.
As for me there'll never ever be another,
That I can love like I love my big brother.

All my love, Forever and Always
Your sister Anne

Chapter 5

Grief without end

In this chapter the wife of a stroke survivor courageously and honestly shares her experience of her family's journey since her husband John suffered a life-changing stroke. In response, Dr Giles Yeates, a brain injury clinician who regularly works with families, offers some thoughts that draw attention to themes throughout Laura's account that connect with key issues in professionals' understanding (or lack of it). In addition, Giles explores how Laura's experiences, common with many other relatives, can stimulate new, much needed directions in the future development of services and awareness of the needs of families following a brain injury.

The story

I had known John at work since 1990. John sadly lost his first wife to breast cancer in 1994, leaving him a single parent with twin boys Daniel and Luke, then aged 5. Several of us at work knew John well, we all travelled back and forth to work together, and supported him during this difficult time. It was at the work Christmas party that we became closer and we began a relationship which could only work if the boys were happy too. Thankfully for us all things worked out and we married in 1999 and then went on to have Ben and then Sophie. John worked in banking and for the last few years was commuting to London. The jobs weren't available locally at that level, so he tended to do about two days at a local office initially and then three in London, and that increased to sort of five in London. Sometimes he would stay overnight, but the bank stopped paying for his overnight accommodation, so he was travelling daily, leaving here about 5 in the morning, getting home at 7 at night. Although a challenge at times with four children of differing needs and ages, we both loved it. Daniel then went onto university and Luke joined the Navy.

It was on the 19th of March 2012 that our lives changed forever.

John had been feeling under the weather for five days beforehand – head and neck pain, and had been taking paracetomol/ibuprofen to help but had been continuing to work, and there was certainly no warning of what was about to come.

The day before was Mother's Day and we'd had a lovely family day, and John had helped Ben and Sophie with their cards and gifts. That evening, after we'd put the children to bed, we were sitting together on the sofa and John said that his neck pain was really bothering him, and that he would take himself off to bed in the spare bedroom, (so as not to disturb me). In hindsight now, this was a bad decision. Had he been in the same bed with me I would have known the timing of his stroke. He kissed me and said goodnight and little did I know that this would be the last time he would say those words to me in our home and walk upstairs – the next time he came down the stairs would be in a chair carried by the paramedics. When I went up to bed later I looked in and checked on John to hear him sound asleep and snoring!

The next morning – Monday 19th March 2012 – I woke as usual with the alarm and got washed and dressed. There was no sound from the spare bedroom so I left John to sleep (or so I thought), whilst I woke Ben for school and came downstairs to start the breakfasts. Ben came on down once he was dressed and I asked him if Dad was up, to which he replied 'No.' This was unusual as John was a light sleeper and by now he would have been woken by the general morning hubbub. I went upstairs to find John on the floor, mumbling, not able to speak or move, and with signs that he'd wet himself. It now appears that he'd woken at some point to visit the bathroom but likely that he'd had a stroke causing him to collapse.

At this point I went into what I can only describe as panic, ran downstairs, told Ben to stay in the dining room eating breakfast, and I ran across to my neighbours, Paul and Lisa. They answered the door and I just cried, 'I think John's had a stroke!' They both came running over, ran upstairs and told me to ring for an ambulance. Paul stayed upstairs talking to John, Lisa sat with Ben and I dialled 999. The call operator kept me talking whilst I waited for the ambulance to arrive, which felt like the last thing I wanted to do – I just wanted to be with John, Ben and Sophie – back to normal – this couldn't be happening. It was probably only a few minutes but felt like forever. Eventually, a paramedic arrived and I took him upstairs to John. Sadly as he got to the top of the stairs, Sophie had woken up, opened her bedroom door and saw the paramedic going into the spare bedroom. I didn't know which way to turn – John? Ben? Or Sophie? He began to assess John and I asked him if John had had a stroke – he didn't answer me – naturally his focus was on John. By this time my mum had arrived too and she kept the children in the dining room to protect them. After 45 minutes an ambulance arrived and John was taken down the stairs in a chair and I prepared to leave with him. Fortunately a friend was able to come in the ambulance with me and I continually kept talking to John, holding his hand, and reassuring him that everything would be ok, despite my obvious distress. How silly that sounds now!

We were blue-lighted to hospital and were greeted by a stroke consultant at A&E. John was taken to be assessed and I was ushered into a small room and there I stayed until the consultant came to tell me they were taking John for a scan. By now I was very upset and distressed – not knowing what was happening – not knowing what the future held. I made a couple of telephone calls. I felt that at some point I would wake up from this nightmare – it was just a haze. After some time the consultant re-appeared to advise that John had a clot on his brain and would be taken up to the stroke unit. We followed him up and at this point John was still able to mumble and I just constantly re-assured him and held him tight. The consultant confirmed that John had had a stroke and advised me that there was very little they could do for him as the clot-busting drugs need to be administered within a few hours, and I was unaware at what time John had his stroke. However, the consultant kept saying 'This man is 50 years old with young children! I'll do all I can to get him across to the local neurological unit to see if they can help in any way.'

At lunchtime, John was finally given the ok to be moved to the neuro-centre – I clearly remember the nurse from ITU at our local hospital explaining how John would be sedated to be moved, and the nurse had a lovely empathic manner about him, and seemed to understand my distress at the whole situation. I was advised to go home and await a call once John had arrived at the specialist unit. By this time my sister had arrived and took us home. Once home, my sister took charge and made me a cup of tea and some lunch. We then received the call and set off. This was a 45-minute journey but seemed to take forever. As soon as we arrived we were ushered into ITU and met by a consultant. They needed my consent to inject dye through the groin up into his brain. I was advised to visit John beforehand as his chances of survival at this point were slim – he was laid on a flat bed in what seemed like a theatre and he was unconscious – I kissed him, told him I loved him and left the room to await the outcome.

The test established he had two blood clots, one had dispersed, one was still there but they were unable to remove it as there was the chance that they could have risked damaging it, so their decision was just to leave things well alone, and just to wait and see how things developed. John was in the neurological unit for about three days, but there was a consultant there, and to this day I can't remember his name, but he was absolutely amazing! And he just said 'I am doing everything I can,' he said, 'I have been pulling people aside in the corridor to say look I have got this man, he is 50, he has got two young children,' and he was the same age, and had three children, and I think it just really hit home. 'If there is anything I have missed, anything else I can do ...' Of course, the answer was no ... The consultant explained in an open, honest but caring way that John's recovery would be 2 to 3 years with severe disabilities, and he sadly was right. I clearly remembered a Scottish nurse in ICU who cried with me when I was told this news.

I really felt that people were going out of their way, and going that extra mile, for John and myself and our family. I can't explain why, because I have never been in that situation before, so you haven't got anything to compare it with, but it really did feel at that moment, those were the two times that I have really felt we had some support.

As soon as I came home that night, the day he had his stroke, from then on, I have always just been constantly open and honest with the children, so everything I was told I would communicate to them on their level, but in a gentle way. It was a heart-breaking conversation to have with them and we hugged and cried together. So when the consultant told me at the neurological unit that John's recovery was going to take two to three years, with severe disabilities, I communicated that fact to them as well, so that they knew I wasn't hiding anything from them. I am always led by the children, their questions and their needs.

John remained in hospital for three days, and he was then transferred back to critical care locally where they kept him stable whilst unconscious. An intensive care unit is a surreal place – very quiet and calm (except the general humming and buzzing of machines), but staff are not rushing about, as you would imagine in an area of critically ill patients.

Within a week they managed to remove his ventilation tubes, so he was breathing independently. And then at that point he was transferred to the stroke unit. I think that was probably one of my worse moments. It was in the old part of the hospital, full of much older people than John, in wards of eight patients, and when they were just wheeling John down the corridor, I just broke down. In fact, I can remember now just turning away, saying 'He is not staying here! He is not staying here!' I just didn't want him in that ward, and I mean the nurses were lovely, but it was dire. Sadly, periodically through the day and night, new patients would arrive, the curtains drawn round, and you could hear the consultants having the same conversation, 'Right can you talk, can you smile?' 'When did this happen? Right, now we can give you this drug, this drug is …' I think two out of three people respond to it, and of course that felt hard as well, because I knew that John wasn't able to have that drug, so that ward felt a pretty dreadful place to be.

It was two weeks after he had his stroke before Ben and Sophie came to visit John. The ward sister from the rehabilitation ward sat down and told them exactly what they were going to see, because he was tube-fed, had oxygen and obviously was nothing like they would have remembered him. It was naturally an upsetting time for us all, but continuing to talk to the children and explaining everything meant that they were less afraid and had my reassurance.

Three weeks later, once a bed became available, John was moved to the rehab ward. This was generally a better place for him to be and the staff were good. The rehab involved physiotherapists, occupational therapists (OTs), speech and language therapy, and a psychologist was there as well, who was helpful for me to speak to from time to time. However, John made little progress, and remained bed bound, tube fed, and without speech. I visited him daily, dropping the children off at school, catching up with things at home, before heading to the hospital, and then back in time for the end of school.

My only criticism of the rehab ward was the review process; the first one was horrendous. They were in a temporary ward, they had had to move because the other one was being decorated, but my sister and I walked in and there was one long table, and all the staff were all sitting facing me, so it was like going for a job interview! I was just in bits when I went home, it was a horrible experience. It was like being put on trial; of course they were also talking about discharge dates, and I was thinking about how I would cope with John at home. This was only two months since he had had his stroke, so I was all over the place. I don't even know if I have come to terms with it now, let alone then. The purpose of the meeting was for all parties to discuss John and communicate their views on his needs but it also felt as though I was being interrogated.

The following day when I went in I spoke to the ward sister and expressed my feelings, which they appreciated, and endeavoured to resolve the issues for future meetings for other families.

Eventually, 7 months after his stroke John was transferred to a long-stay, slow-stream neuro rehabilitation home. John had physio, OT and speech and language sessions, and within a year he progressed to being able to sit in a wheelchair, began to speak, managed to eat a soft diet, and eventually had his PEG line (his feeding tube) removed. He remained there for 2 years, after which he was moved to the adjacent bungalow where he still resides today. It's a much smaller home with five residents, a caring, friendly, welcoming environment, generally a nice space for us to visit and be together as a family. It is our preferred long-term care plan for him but unfortunately there is no certainty. John is right-side affected, and remains wheelchair bound, doubly incontinent – he does not have the cognition to be able to initiate any speech or actions but generally responds when spoken to. He has very passive behaviour which can be a challenge as it is difficult at times to establish his needs, and he is totally dependent on others. When people ask me how he is, I reply 'He's well-cared for, and happy and content enough.' Can I, as his wife, really ask for more than that?

The majority of the staff there are great, and the MDT have been an immense support to us. I have had issues along the way, but I tend to raise them at the time or maybe a bit later with the key worker. The hardest bit for me has been the continuing health care fight, which started in June 2013. This is when they decided they needed to do an assessment to see if John qualified for Continuing Health Care funding (CHC).

Nobody ever explained to me how the process would work and what was involved in the assessment. How useful it would have been to supply families with a leaflet or documentation to explain the steps and projected timescale of the process. It is very clinical, form-led, and in our case, I was treated as an outsider and felt disregarded, whilst the clinical professionals discuss your loved one around you. The health professionals naturally use medical terminology, a language which I very quickly learnt to enable me to understand the system and processes.

There was a lady there from CHC, who was dreadful. Halfway through the meeting, she turned around to me and said sorry, what was your name again? Even though we had all introduced ourselves. She asked me why I wasn't having John back at home, which of course makes me feel guilty, even now, and I know it is not the right thing to do for him. I don't think we could cope and things would be very different if he was at home. So that was an awful experience. They did the first assessment in October 2013, during which the MDT agreed he should qualify for funding. The assessor again, the same lady, was just awful, arguing every point, and downgrading each of John's abilities a level, so of course consequently when it went to the panel, they didn't agree funding. Rather than putting in an appeal, I lodged a complaint with the Care Commissioning Group (CCG), against the way the process had been done as it had not been conducted in accordance with the national framework rules. I even contacted our local MP for support, and to express my disgust at the handling of the process.

I have always documented issues regarding John and his care, so I had plenty of evidence to back up his case, and with the help and support of my sister, we wrote a six-page letter. About 2 months later, I received their reply – no apologies, just confirming their position and advising that if I wanted to take things further to arrange a meeting with them. In June 2014 we met up with the Director of Quality at the CCG – she was a breath of fresh air because I felt she was listening to me, and seemed to understand my grievances. She agreed there were many issues with their handling of John's case. The nurse assessor had even wanted to meet with a lady from the nursing home to hand over John's notes at Marks and Spencers – this was absolutely inappropriate. She was appalled by many things that had happened, and so she asked me what I would like to happen. She couldn't guarantee the assessment decision would change, but I decided I would like the assessment redone, and even if it were to turn out negatively, at least I would know in my heart that it had been done properly and that I had fought for John.

The second assessment was carried out in August 2014. I heard in December it had gone to panel, and they had agreed six months rehab funding. We were all dismayed … even the social worker; the social worker actually is another person who has been amazing, a young lady who just really understands and gets it. Just six months rehab funding. John had not been on a rehab programme for 18 months, he had rehab input for the first 6 months, and then they downgraded it to a maintenance package due to his lack of improvement. And then unbeknown to everybody else, it was revisited by panel the following week where they finally agreed he was eligible for CHC funding. This process now gets reviewed on an annual basis.

It has been a battle that I never would have envisaged, and at times when I look back, I cannot believe I got through it. There have been times, though, that I have literally been on the floor, unable to put up this fight anymore, together with mourning the loss of my husband. But somehow, something inside gets you through. If I had fallen at the first hurdle, we would not have achieved the level of care that John needs and is receiving now.

The reality

Why us? Why now? John had just turned 50 and we'd had such a lovely holiday away for Christmas and the New Year. It was the first time we'd spent Christmas away from home and we felt free of the day to day drudges sitting in the sunshine. The older boys were now 23 and much older, living independently and settled in their lives. Ben and Sophie too were growing up, now 11 and 8, and less dependent, which made it much easier for us all to go away. It was also becoming time for John and me to spend together because when we got together he had the boys and, after marrying, we then went on to have Ben and Sophie. We both deeply enjoyed being parents and having a family unit, but had had very little time alone – this was something we were both looking forward to in the future.

The hardest thing is to stop feeling guilty.

It's hard to laugh or have fun without feeling guilty and for that laughter to be proper pure happiness. It's always tinged with sadness but as time moves on the laughter begins to recover. It's taken a long time to learn to laugh again and to laugh and feel that that's ok because, ultimately, I owe it to myself – it's my life. I have to live my life. What's the point of continuing year after year wallowing, feeling sad, it doesn't help me, it doesn't help John and certainly doesn't help the children. But how do you move forward and live your life when you're constantly pulled back into the situation you're in on a daily basis, whether you want to be or not?

Mine is an ongoing grief – an 'ambiguous loss' – this is one of the most difficult feelings to manage on a daily basis. It never leaves you no matter how hard you try to move forward. But each day, you wake up, put on your 'face', hold your head up, smile, and carry on with life, whilst always carrying the load or baggage that cannot be left behind. It is very hard to remain positive and drive yourself forward; however, probably having some inbuilt strong core values is what has kept me going. I also find it's much easier to be strong and fight when you are doing it for somebody else, so when, for example, I was fighting for John's funding or there was an issue with him or perhaps he wasn't being cared for properly, no problem, I could go in and voice my opinion and get things sorted. Likewise for the children – if they had a problem at school, I could go into the school and sort it out. However, if it is something directly for me it's a different story.

Something I always wanted was to be heard or listened to. I do NOT want sympathy but just a degree of empathy and support by people trying their best to understand the situation I was in and why I was behaving in a certain way.

How difficult it is watching carers take care of John, (my husband), and being told of his likes and dislikes. I know what he likes – I'm his wife. I cannot be with him all the time but on the times I am with him, please listen to me. On one particular occasion John had a headache – the carer told me John loves to have his head massaged and then proceeded to tip his wheelchair back and massage his face and head. This was great for John but for me, as a wife, watching on as another woman caresses his head, it was difficult. I'm his wife – do I not count? There comes a point when you have to accept and step back from these emotional situations. Fighting for his daily needs is not easy and maybe I don't know what's best for him now and maybe those that are caring for him on a daily basis do; however, I still think there's some deep-rooted bond between John and myself whereby we probably know each other better than anyone else knows each of us.

It is heartbreaking watching other families out and about having fun. Weekends or holidays are particularly difficult for me, maybe not so much for the children. Seeing other couples too having a closeness or neighbours out for a walk hand-in-hand. It is totally normal and acceptable for me to see, it is just another reminder of what I have lost and don't have anymore. It isn't fair.

One year, John's care home held a New Year's Eve party, with a DJ, for all the residents and their families, on December 30th at 5 p.m. The three of us went along, and afterwards Ben and Sophie said 'It was great Mum! We had a lovely time and thank you for taking us.' One minute I just thought, What am I doing here? And the next I realised this is our life now. Two very different realities.

I am learning to appreciate what I've got. I am lucky to be where I am – I have amazing children and I am thankful for that. Sometimes I live life taking one day at a time or even one hour at a time just to be able to move forward. Whatever my situation there will always be someone worse off than me. But how do I accept that this is now my life? Living in limbo. Frozen in time. Life moves on but I'm not moving on with it.

The constant feeling of being alone is particularly hard at the end of the day when all you want to do is sit down on the sofa and sound off at somebody or just for someone else to listen to your day, what has happened, the frustrations of being a parent, etc. It is not easy to deal with this on your own. I think it's a natural human instinct to want to share and bond with somebody and have some closeness, or just a hug at the end of the day would be enough. But that's gone.

I have constant frustrations when something goes wrong within the house or with technology etc., particularly if I can't rectify it myself. It means calling someone in and sometimes paying a professional to sort things out. Often this is a tipping point for my emotions – I have no-one else to call on – I have to step up to the mark.

Why do people watch us when we're out as family with John? We're just trying to be a normal family unit. It's difficult enough going out with John without people looking and staring. Particularly hard for the children when that happens. It even happened in hospital – in the place you'd least expect it people to look and stare but they still did!

It is now my role to manage the emotions of the family – this can change on a daily basis or even hour by hour, and is particularly difficult at significant family events when our losses are felt even more strongly and we're pulled right back emotionally to where we were despite trying to move forward. The nature of having children is that their lives are constantly moving forward and moving on as they progress through the school years. This is a natural progression for any child; however, at times we are pulled right back, and the pain is felt at that point. As Ben quite rightly said, 'It's just like something is permanently missing from home, Mum.'

Our friends have dwindled away. All those people who were there right from the start – a constant stream of texts, phone calls, cards, letters – slowly after about 6 months this stopped. People seem to think that after a period of time you are coping and what people see from the outside is not necessarily what is going on in the inside. People don't know what to say or how to behave and so they behave in a way that they think is best for me, rather than asking me what I need. Although actually it is very often difficult for me to know what I need or would like.

I never envisaged bringing up our children alone, it is not the environment I would have wished for them to grow up in. However, they have grown into amazing people who are well-rounded and have a deep appreciation for mental and physical disabilities.

It is very difficult when I knew John better than anyone else, as he did me, after being together for 16 years prior to his stroke. We both knew each other's plans/thoughts better than anyone else, as you would within a relationship/marriage, but sadly this has been challenged in various ways since his stroke, as he does not have the mental capacity to voice his own opinion.

I have learnt over the years, when people ask me how I am, to just reply 'I'm fine,' as people are generally not interested to hear how you really are, and if I do explain, they don't know how to respond.

I think I probably channelled all my grief, anger, frustration, emotions, into fighting for the best possible care and funding for John. It was a case of getting what he was entitled to for his needs. This kept my mind occupied together with bringing up the children, supporting Daniel and Luke, and managing the house and finances, rather than allowing myself time to grieve. The grieving process probably began once I was over this huge hurdle, and is an ongoing process. There are good days and bad days, days of positivity and days of despair. Rather like a hilly walk – many ups and downs! Anniversaries, birthdays, Christmas, or other special occasions or moments of achievement for the children, are all particularly difficult times to cope with, as it just highlights the fact that John is missing. Physically he is still here (not at home), but mentally he is not. I try to remember the good times but it is not easy when today's reality is so very different.

Does John still recognise me? Yes he does. Do I still recognise him? Now, that's a different question altogether. Physically, the man I see sitting in his wheelchair is still the man I married. However, his responses to me and the children at times, are very much removed from who he was before his stroke. I sometimes find myself just looking at him looking into his eyes, trying to get a glimpse of what is going on in his head – what he is thinking or feeling – but it just draws a blank – a sense of nothingness. I cannot put into words how this feels, and sometimes he feels like a stranger and yet physically he is there. And yet he looks at me as if nothing has changed.

There have been very few areas of support for us as a family as we are in a unique group. A brain-injured husband/father who lives in a residential nursing home. The Stroke Association was my first point of contact, but they generally supported the elderly. Different Strokes is a very good charity supporting younger stroke victims and their families; however, their help for us was limited as John was not living at home. Headway is a great charity for brain-injured people and their families but when the family meetings are held, they take along their brain-injured loved one, which I was unable to do. Kids (young carers), is another fantastic charity supporting young people who are caring for a loved one, and whilst Ben and Sophie care for their Dad when they visit him at the weekend, it is not full-time, and they felt like they didn't fit in. Simon Says is an amazing bereavement charity for bereaved children, and whilst Ben and Sophie are grieving in a similar way, it is not suitable for them. We feel quite alone with our grief.

The feedback that I have received from the MDT is how much they have learnt from us as a family, through my drive to fight for John, and from the way the children have conducted themselves in a nursing home environment and around their Dad. I would like to hope that the Continuing Health Care team have learnt from their errors and misdemeanours; however, sadly I am not sure this has been the case. Even following on from my complaint to the Care Commissioning Group, the promises they made have not been carried out. This situation does cause you to question and lose trust in the health care professionals.

My advice to anyone in an unfortunate similar situation would be to fight for what you believe in and not to be coerced into making any decisions that you don't feel comfortable with. Always go with your gut instinct, as that generally is the right one to go with. To have a professional or advocate alongside me from the start, to support and guide me through the many challenges along the way, would have been a blessing, but sadly this is not something that is provided or even considered by the NHS.

I still love John but I am no longer in love with him. I wish someone had told me that it was ok for me to feel this way, it would have given me more peace of mind. It has been very difficult coming to terms with this change in my feelings. I have strong core values, which have helped me get through to here.

I have gradually reduced the frequency of my visits to John to twice a week. It has taken me several years to have the reassurance and confidence in knowing that he's cared for well enough whether I am visiting or not, and that he is happy and content enough. He is unable to remember whether I have visited and I am gradually learning to put the guilt I feel when I am not there, into a little box and close the lid.

My coping mechanism when making tough decisions is now to just go with my gut instinct at the time, and not to overthink it or worry what others may say. It may not be the right decision a week later, but at the original time and place it was my gut instinct and that's ok.

The bitterness I feel when people see me and the first thing they ask is 'How is John?'! Naturally, I understand that is and always will be the focus, and what has happened to him has taken his life (as we knew it), away. But he is ok, he's safe, well-cared for, and happy and content enough. But what about me? This little person who feels insignificant but is the one person holding the family together – bringing up two children amongst these uncertainties – caring for John – managing the house and garden – managing the finances, etc. It's like I am on autopilot! I often can't remember yesterday, am often not living today, but am constantly thinking about what's happening tomorrow. I should be living in the moment but sometimes that's too painful.

Be kind to yourself.

Giles Yeates' response to Laura's account

When I read Laura's account, I was both gripped by her evocative clarity and articulation of complex experiences, and also struggled with the feelings of discomfort that it brought. I read this during some time off from my clinical work; I could hear my wife and children in the house downstairs, my expectations of life intact and proceeding as intended. In my clinical work and professional writing, I strive to increase professional and public awareness of many of the issues powerfully communicated by Laura. However, when it is there, expressed so directly as in Laura's account, it was hard to take in as a process of complete witnessing. I cannot begin to imagine how it is to be in the epicentre of these experiences. However, I will try and open a conversation with Laura from the professional's perspective, linking key themes in her account to both the clinical literature and the stories of other relatives and survivors that I encounter often in my work. I have focused on the three themes of relationships versus individuals; professional responses to the complex and enduring needs of survivors and their loved ones, and the process of recognising each other in the family post-injury.

Inter-connection in relationships following brain injury versus isolated (and ignored) individuals

Laura's account of couples and family life before the stroke, in its aftermath and during the evolution of time through the present and into the future paints a vivid and moving picture of the brain injury as a relational event. That is, a wave that was created by the ischaemic lesion of the stroke in John's brain, as a boulder impacts on a lake, followed by a ripple that picks up mass and turns into a wave that not only disables John's mind but passes through all those who are connected to, and love John, compromising their feelings, minds, and sense of connection with John. This wave also extends through time, as Laura describes. Rather than family challenges getting easier, being static, or resolving themselves with the supposed healing passing of time, each milestone in a family member's life is defined by the absence of John as his pre-stroke self – a husband to Laura, a father to Daniel, Luke, Ben and Sophie.

Laura's account also highlights how this essential relational dimension of stroke and other brain injuries, this impact on and between all those connected to a survivor, can be missed by the various professionals that the family encounter on their journey post-injury. All attention is focused on the boulder, not the wave, drawn inward to the level of brain tissue and ignoring the web of shattered and strained human relationships around the survivor. The widening impact of the ripple was also evident in Laura's sense that family friends dwindled away over time – progressive social isolation for survivors and their immediate families has been repeatedly demonstrated in the literature (Elsass and Kinsella, 1987). Services are usually focused around the survivor, needs are conceptualised with the skull as a limiting boundary (Bowen et al., 2010, Yeates, 2007). Relatives are invited to meetings about the survivor, with relatives' own distress often an uncomfortable phenomenon that professional's feel ill-equipped to respond to. Services may stretch to offering relatives groups, rarer still whole-family sessions. Professionals focused on the needs of survivors (which they can find overwhelming at even the individual level, see next section) often automatically partition off the experience of relatives (the professional perspective severing and masking the interconnection of such to that of the survivor) and as a result do not engage with relatives in a responsive, compassionate way (the behaviour of the CHC representative in Laura's account is a good example of this).

Reluctance of statutory services to acknowledge complex and enduring nature of ABI

I was really struck, saddened and moved by Laura's account of her repeated interactions with the CHC representative. Unfortunately, this is an all too common scenario. Another striking example can be found in the book *Where Is the Mango Princess?* by Cathy Crimmins (Crimmins, 2001), the wife of a traumatic brain injury survivor. Her brutally honest narrative retells the journey of a family both pulled apart by the brain injury and then having to negotiate contrasting health care systems (and funding responses) of Canada and the USA during the subsequent weeks and months.

The long-term and complex nature of brain injury consequences has been established in the scientific literature and public awareness of the big picture is also growing. New research only widens the scope of post-injury difficulties day by day. So the question then emerges: why is there a constant struggle to persuade commissioners, social services and some brain injury services themselves to also acknowledge this reality and start (and remain) on the same page as survivors and families? It is my personal belief that the reality is just too overwhelming for those professionals whose role it is to allocate ongoing funds and create service models to support post-injury needs. It is telling that one relevant document, the Department of Health's *National Service Framework for Long Term (Neurological) Conditions* (NSF-LT(n)C) did acknowledge the long-term reality of post-injury support needs and set out a Quality Requirement that all specialist brain injury services adopt a life-span approach (Department of Health, 2005). That is, build capacity to be there for survivors and their families in the years and decades post-injury as they and their families encounter long-term challenges. While this government paper set this requirement out in black and white, the document has subsequently been a far less potent influence than initially envisaged – NHS brain injury community services continue in the main to offer time-limited provision only, and funds have to be fought for, sometimes repeatedly (be this health commissioners, social care budgets, Department of Work and Pensions benefits, medico-legal settlements). The words of the NSF-LT(n)C have either been forgotten, never consulted or ignored. Beyond resource capacity issues, I do also feel there is an emotional dynamic at play, where the pain and hardship experienced by survivors and their families threatens to overwhelm professionals if they let it in. What is increasingly problematic is that the (progressively) myopic remits of services result in the perspectives of professionals working in those services becoming increasingly adrift from those in survivors' personal lives – clinicians just passing through at discrete moments while the long-term nature of brain injury continues to unfold following discharge. Laura notes both the important role of third sector organisations such as Different Strokes and Headway alongside health care providers, but also the limitations of these groups. The necessity for professionals to be available for the long haul and walk alongside survivors and their loved ones is paramount.

Recognition of familiar selves following brain injuries

One of the most complicated tasks faced by the families is to recognise and maintain the identity of survivor in the years post-injury. It is clear that in this case each family member had their unique thread of recognition with their husband or father, that was uniquely theirs to share with John within each particular relationship in the family. Laura describes how she knew him better than anyone else in the world, as he knew her. She explores how she felt familiar to John, but how she experienced a complex set of feelings in response to the uncertainty of his gaze on her and the possibility of nothingness in certain moments. This juxtaposition of familiarity, recognition and alienation are central challenges to the psychological connections between people following brain injury. However, these experiences are so complicated and hard to express to others, and have not been adequately explored in the literature (with the rare exception of Pauline Boss's work on Ambiguous Loss and partner accounts of their experiences, such as Cathy Crimmins' aforementioned book and an article by Feigelson, who is both a wife of a brain injury survivor and a psychoanalyst [Feigelson, 1993]).

It must have been so strange, unreal and maddening to see well-meaning professionals describe their own sense of John's wishes, intentions and preferences, having never known him before. I often reflect on this in my work, how for the most part I enter the lives of a survivor and their family post-injury, and how this puts me on a completely different page to the people I support. I do feel that it can be emancipatory for myself and the survivor, as it allows us to create a psychological road forward that is free of the historical constraints and painful contradictions that others in the survivor's family struggle with. Yet, this new possibility must always be tempered with a need to be orientated to the intimacy of immediate family knowledge and recognition of each other across time, in a way not discernible to strangers or even the wider family. Without attempting to find out about these perspectives behind closed doors, professionals will never be able to approach the pain experienced when these bonds have been strained or severed.

Summary

Laura's account included three painful dimensions of a family's struggle following a life-changing stroke: the impact of the injury on relationships (not just one brain); the enduring and complex nature of needs for both the survivor and their loved ones (and the struggle to get professionals and agencies on the same page as those experiencing these needs), and the challenge of recognising one another post-injury, amidst the necessary but unwanted presence of strangers in the post-injury life of John and his family. These themes have been noted in the professional literature before, but it is important for the immediacy of subjective perspectives held by those affected by these issues to be constantly and forcefully retold. In this way, as uncomfortable as it can be to read, professionals involved in supporting survivors and families are more likely to hold an awareness and sensitivity to these needs that may make them more responsive and useful to the people they support. This awareness is always vulnerable to losing its intensity within the procedures of professional practice, so accounts such as Laura's are welcome, important and necessary to re-sensitise and reprioritise these themes in the minds of professionals. I hope too, that this account adds to others that make other survivors and relatives feel validated and less alone in their experiences, as they also struggle with these too common challenges.

References

Bowen, C., Yeates, G., & Palmer, S.O.N. 2010. *A relational approach to rehabilitation: thinking about relationships after brain injury.* London: Karnac.

Crimmins, C. 2001. *Where is the Mango Princess?: a journey back from brain injury.* New York: Random House Digital.

Department of Health 2005. *National service framework for long-term conditions.* London: DoH.

Elsass, L., & Kinsella, G. 1987. Social interaction following severe closed head injury. *Psychological Medicine*, 17, 67–78.

Feigelson, C. 1993. Personality death, object loss, and the uncanny. *International Journal of Psycho-analysis*, 74, 331.

Yeates, G. 2007. Avoiding the skull seduction in post-acute acquired brain injury services: individualist invitations and systemic responses. *Clinical Psychology Forum* (British Psychological Society) N.S., 175, 33–36.

Chapter 6

Support of siblings

Introduction

When I (Jo Clark-Wilson) was working as an occupational therapist as a member of a multidisciplinary team in acute and long-term brain injury rehabilitation units 30 years ago, we took all opportunities to see a patient's relatives, as and when they visited, to aid the patient's transition home. The specialist units were usually situated a distance from the patient's home and outreach services to support community integration were not easy to find. The experienced social worker was usually involved to support the patient's discharge home or to their next placement. At that time, professionals had limited understanding and experience of working with the severely brain injured population, let alone their families. When reflecting on this, I believe I had a short-sighted, short-term view and do not think the multidisciplinary team really considered, understood or properly supported and addressed the families' needs at this time.

Only on becoming a brain injury case manager and working in community settings did the full impact of 'brain injury' on relatives and overall family functioning over time become so evident that my clinical practice and approach changed. I am grateful to all the clients and families who allowed me into their lives to work with them, as they helped me gain greater appreciation and understanding of the issues that affected them and invaluable skills to help me support others.

It is acknowledged that everyone is different and what works for one person and family does not necessarily work for another. I have learnt that if the individual with the brain injury is not considered within the context of their family, with full collaboration for developing the ways forward, many therapeutic interventions are unsuccessful in the community. Our role is to listen without judgement, be honest and focused, create ideas, support what will be helpful, work at the family's pace and 'be there for them'.

Investigating the issues

In the next two chapters, I have focused on the reflections of two siblings and three children, all of whom have relatives, who sustained very
severe brain injuries in accidents over 25 years ago. I am, or was,
actively involved as a case manager for their parent/sibling for many
years, so I have some knowledge and experience of the issues that arose
during that time.

The relatives were asked whether they would be willing to share their
perspectives and reflections, to find out:

- the impact of their relatives' brain injury on their life;
- the changes in roles and relationships that occurred as a consequence, not only with their injured relative but also with other
  members of family and their friends;
- any stories/reflections of situations that occurred which were of
  significance to them;
- anything they believed made a difference to them;
- whether they had a message that might help other children/
  siblings.

I share their personal stories with you and am grateful to them for
their open and honest communication and transparency of feelings. I
picked out the themes from their narratives and my comments on their
reflections are only included, if relevant, to highlight other information
that can add value to their stories. All people have been anonymised,
so it is not possible to identify those with the brain injury.

In reviewing their personal stories from over 25 years, there was
some information given that I had not fully appreciated at the time,
which gave me new perspectives and understanding. Of most significance was the emotional content of their narrative. This struck a
chord with me, as I could appreciate the scenarios from their perspective; but also, on occasions, feel the discordance and unease, when I
recalled the conflicts that I, as a case manager, had struggled to
address so many years earlier. It provided an up-to-date review and it
was fascinating for me to read and understand how they felt they had
coped with ongoing issues over time.

Eliza and Frances

Two siblings were approached to see if they felt comfortable sharing
their reflections and experiences over so many years. Whilst I had

worked with their injured relative and parents for over 25 years, I had less contact with these siblings. Their stories were shared via telephone interviews.

The first story is of Eliza, who was in her late teens when her younger sister Frances (both of whom were adopted) sustained a severe brain injury in a road traffic accident. Frances was aged 17. Eliza's parents provided care for Frances in their home for the following 9 years without any assistance, apart from occasional visits from a Social Worker. Eliza's parents supported Frances to move into her own flat nearby on two occasions, but she could not manage independently, flooded the flat and had to return to the parental home. When I first became involved it was clear that Frances lacked insight, had poor executive functioning, high levels of anxiety and agitation, and limited appreciation of risks. She was highly responsive to negative influences in her environment. Eliza's parents were under extreme stress due to Frances' behaviour towards them (constant unreasonable demands, directed verbal abuse, and control of their environment). Frances moved out again, this time with additional input from support workers, but this care regime also broke down. She was admitted, under Section, to a specialist unit for rehabilitation. Further attempts have been made since then to support Frances in a specialist residential setting, a community group home and in her own home with varying degrees of support, but nothing has proved permanently successful to date.

I only really met Eliza as her parents grew older. Eliza started to attend case conferences at the specialist unit Frances was residing in and gradually, over time, became more involved in the care regime for her sister. After Eliza's parents died, within five days of each other about three years ago, she took over their roles in supporting Frances.

Eliza described Frances' life before and directly after the accident.

> Frances and I were adopted. As a child my sister had romantic ideas and loved film stars. I was the quiet one. When Frances was a youngster, she always pushed the boundaries. She was always in trouble at school. She was wild and headstrong – would stay out – cause a lot of grief for my parents – everything she could do, she did. At 17 she talked about drinking, smoking marijuana and having access to drugs. She left home a couple of times – my parents were always consistent and, whatever she did, they always looked after her. My parents got behind her and guided her in the right direction and, at the time of the accident, she was due to start a new job.

I had left home and been married for about a year when my sister's accident occurred. I remember the night it happened. In ICU, just after the accident, mum was told by a nurse, 'Pray she dies.' They did not understand this at the time, but mum found out later. She did not know when my sister emerged from coma, she would not be the same – it took her a long time to recognise that.

I was halfway through studying on a course, but had to give this up, as I was visiting my sister and supporting mum, so I got behind in my work. After having my children, I did further study when my daughter was young, so it did not affect my future in the long term.

Life changed over the years – initially there was all the hospital visits and then when Frances went home (to the care of my parents), it was intense. It was my mum really who bore the brunt of it. Frances took everything from my mum and there were lots of run-ins with my dad, which I tried to avoid. Then Frances lived in a house up the road and when this broke down, she went away for rehabilitation. When Frances moved away, the focus was still there but just not on our doorstep.

Eliza discussed the impact Frances's accident had on the family unit, particularly on her parents.

It affected our relationship as a family for a period of time afterwards. I felt pushed out. I visited them, but it was always a bit strained, as my sister was so volatile. Everyone had to stand to her tune and everyone tiptoed around her to keep the peace. Tension all the time and she always had to air her issues.

I felt resentful for a period of time, as all the attention was focused on her. My sister was always the topic of conversation. My mum was burdening herself and we could not have a normal conversation. Then I talked to my mum about it and it helped. Mum always did her very best to support us both. When my son was born, my mum came around every day. Over time that feeling of resentment left me and I understood my sister a bit better.

I was support for my mum rather than my dad, as he never really understood. Dad could not talk about anything. Even when he and mum were poorly, and mum was bedridden, he could not go to her, as he was frightened. I knew that, but I felt guilty as I could not reconcile this, because of the way he behaved towards my mum.

> **Box 6.1 Professional reflection: relationships with family**
>
> I had a very close working alliance with Eliza's mother over a long period of time and am aware how difficult her life was and how much she relied on Eliza for support. Eliza's mother was forever supportive of Frances, even when she was under significant pressure and very ill. On one occasion Eliza's mother informed me she was going to be admitted to hospital for a week, as she had a lump on her breast that required investigation. She had previously suffered from breast cancer. She was looking forward to having a break from caring for Frances. Eliza's mother also commented on one occasion that she would have had a divorce from her husband, if I had not been around. She explained how her husband had never understood Frances' behaviour and treated her like a naughty child rather than acknowledging the problems were a consequence of her brain injury. In a conversation with Eliza's mother about a year before she died, she commented, 'You get tired of it – the older we are the more tired we get and all we want, is to see her (Frances) happy and settled, and when we are not here, there is always Eliza, who is very understanding of Frances' needs and her Case Manager.'

I think initially after mum died, I felt overwhelmed, it seemed like a massive thing that dropped on my lap. My sister used to ring my mum at set times every day or my mum rang her. I cannot not answer the telephone (her mother also had to respond to any telephone calls), I know how my mother felt now.

Eliza described the relationship she has with her sister now.

I battle – but that is me. My sister is sometimes really unhappy and other times she is quite happy in her world doing what she is doing. Frances acts like a child and thinks she cannot be told – her logic is not there any longer – that is the biggest thing – her thought processes are logical to her but not to other people.

I feel guilty as I do not spend enough time with her. I feel guilty as I find her very difficult. I wish I could be more patient with her. I hear the same things over and over again. I have the constant-ness in my ear all the time. When I go out in the car with her or away with her somewhere unfamiliar, she talks to me all the time, telling me the same thing over and over again. I want to say, 'Will you shut up, I'm trying to keep my eyes on the road.' She does not pick up the subtleties of how to act – she does not have that insight.

It is easier for me to go up there and it is ok to be with her for a short period of time. She struggles to sleep when she is staying here with me. We do activities. I take her to concerts. A frustration is she could do so many things, she has the money to do it but all she wants to do is watch television.

I would like to do more and take her to America on my own for a week, but I am unable to manage. We went to Amsterdam and one night was enough. I have to be with her all the time. I cannot leave her to her own devices, as she is easily disoriented. I feel drained. She does not really want to go away. She likes her routines.

However, even now, I have to check myself and remember she has a brain injury. She can't reason. I ask myself, 'Why can't you see that and then realise, "no she can't do it."'

Eliza discussed Frances' relationship with her own family.

To be honest, I struggle with it more than the others in my family, they take her in their stride. They do not see her that much. There was an incident the Christmas after my parents died. I had been with her to buy presents, wrapped them for her and made it feel a bit special, for me rather than her, as she does not care. My kids bought her a present, which I was pleased about. Frances did not like the chocolates and, she cannot help it, whatever is in her head she has to say. After a couple of hours, the children all disappeared. I was upset with her, as she was making comments about my children. I have reflected and stopped beating myself up and we have not bought presents for each other for the past couple of years.

Whilst it was quite a trial when she did come down for Christmas, I still felt guilty when she then decided not to come to stay. She said to me do you mind if I don't come? I agreed that it was important for her to do what she wanted to do, it works better to do this rather than force the issue about Christmas. In any case, I cook a dinner and she covers it in ketchup and mayonnaise and she is not bothered about presents. Frances makes a big deal about being happy watching the television and she gets frustrated if she does not watch what she wants to watch.

Box 6.2 Professional reflection: differences in outlook

Eliza highlighted how she believed she should act as a sister for Frances, for instance, taking her out, spending Christmases together, going on holiday, etc., all of which are shared family values. When Eliza took over from her parents, she believed these were ways of supporting Frances and giving her a better quality of life. In the conversation Eliza acknowledged the discrepancies of these views with those of her sister, who wanted to watch television, stay at home for Christmas and did not want to go away on holiday, as she liked her everyday set routines.

Eliza described how she and Frances were adopted by her parents, and shared her experiences about a situation that occurred after Frances' accident.

After the accident my mum had a letter from my blood relative (sister) to say that the woman who brought me into the world wanted to make contact with me. I met her and my three sisters. I had a kind of romantic feeling of what it would be like but, in fact, it was not like that at all. My adopted mum was my 'mum' and this other one is not my mum. I get on with my sisters and have contact but Frances is my sister, and nothing will change that. I felt I had lost my sister after the accident, but I do not feel like that now.

Eliza was asked what her message for others would be, if they were in a similar situation to herself and she said,

Be accepting of them, as this is who they are, and they are not choosing to be the way they are. Whatever I say or do – she will be the same.

I tried to make her fit in the family mould, for instance, coming to me for Christmas after our parents died. She cannot be moulded – she is happier doing her own thing at Christmas (alone in her flat watching television). My mum would have been mortified.

I try to be the person on her side, even though this is through gritted teeth, at times. Protect yourself too.

Grace and Henry

The second sibling, Grace, was very involved from the early days after her elder brother Henry's accident, in supporting him and her widowed mother Isobel. Henry was in his mid-20s and lived independently of his family when he had his accident. Since his discharge from hospital he has lived with, and been cared for by Isobel with the support of his sibling (Grace) and her family. Grace was the main communicator initially but, due to her own changed personal circumstances, this changed. Now I work more directly with Henry and Isobel, although Grace continues to be actively involved in supporting her mother and brother. These are Grace's recollections:

> My brother is four years older than me. I remember when Henry had the accident. I left my flat and drove to my mother's house in the middle of the night – thinking about him and feeling shocked. I remember stopping at a petrol station to buy a packet of cigarettes, even though I had given up.
>
> After the accident happened, we went into emergency mode – at the hospital – we were 'in a vacuum and nothing was real'. When I went up there on the second night – there were not many staff – it was quiet – it felt unreal and we were in limbo. We sat around watching him and holding his hand, talking to him and to each other. The nurse said he would probably not make it through the night. I was profoundly shocked by how injured he was. I did not know how he could be so damaged and live. But we felt he would – there was a powerful life force and energy – his whole body was vibrating – but yet it also felt as if he was in panic, fearful, fighting for his life. This had a profound impact on me and made me feel really protective.
>
> We visited him every day. At the end of the second week I was sitting by his bedside and was suddenly overwhelmed by a weird, horrible smell. I opened the cupboard door and took a bag out to find out what was in it and found it was all his clothes and shoes they had cut off him after the accident, covered in stuff and saturated with blood. That really shocked me – stuffed in a bag in a locker and not told about it – just left to find it. It felt like he was already written off and did not matter.
>
> A few days after the accident, I went to the site of the crash and I found Henry's business cards and cassettes scattered around the area. I found that really difficult – it did not feel right for aspects of his life to be strewn around the area, and I could not leave it there. I remember feeling emotional – with a sadness his life was over, but he was not dead – and it felt like he had gone and was not coming back.
>
> Henry was moved to a hospital which was more local to where we lived. At this time his head was shaved, he had a huge scar around his head with stitches and was very bruised. But he was mobile. He remembered where the bus station was, got a bus, walked four miles and turned up at home. The hospital rang to say he was missing only after he had arrived home. It was distressing

to see how confused and afraid he was, and terrified by hallu-
cinations. He did not want to go back but they said he needed to
be there, so I took him back, but I felt terrible. I felt I was
abandoning him, as that was his perception. There was no rehab
available to him and shortly afterwards they discharged him into
our care, as they could not manage him, and then the real fun
began. From that time on we were running to catch up – without
time to think or work it out – firefighting – we worried about
missing opportunities for him to make a better recovery – as we
did not know what we were doing. No-one told us what we should
be doing and there was no help or support from anyone.

I stayed at my mother's house to support initially, going back to
my flat as and when to get my stuff. I never returned to my flat. At
that time, Henry was not himself at all – he was frightened, physically aggressive, hallucinating, and very paranoid. He was
unpredictable and could lash out. I was worried sick about leaving
mum alone with him and rang her during the day to confirm she
was all right. We did not get any advice – apart from that most of
the improvements would happen in the first two years, that we
should try and get him to do jigsaws or crosswords to stimulate
him, and that his memory would come back a little more. Professionals were not there – we wanted support. We were lost, as we
did not know what to do – and we did not have access to any
specialist knowledge or guidance. We were making it up as we
went along in a weird sort of bubble. Mum was following her
instincts – she gained an understanding of the psychological and
emotional aspects of him and how he was – and how to work with
him and I followed her lead. Over time I developed my own
instincts about things, as I had a different perspective from
attending medical appointments and we shared these insights
together and from that we pulled out what was best to do. We
looked at his needs – freedom, independence and safety – those
being his most important requirements – and this is why we did
what we did to keep him out of an institution.

We could not make plans for the future, as we did not know if
his current state was a temporary or long-term issue – we did not
know if he was always going to be so difficult to manage or what
was going to happen. With other conditions, like Parkinson's, you
can get information and have an idea of what is going to happen;
with head injury – nothing. We spent many years working out how
to manage him and how to meet his needs and that goes through
changes over time, it's never set.

In the immediate aftermath of the accident I was working flex-
itime and had to juggle my work with hospital visits, appointments
and managing his affairs, etc., so I was often working late at night
to make up time. I then changed my workplace and took a second
job to help financially support the situation.

Then there was the litigation process. The litigation swallowed
up my life for nine years. I do not know where we would be without that money or what life would have been like. The main focus
of those years was getting into court with the strongest case possible to secure his future. Henry's disabilities are not immediately
obvious – the medical experts took him at face value. They were
not listening to us – it is immensely frustrating not being listened
to. There were discrepancies in the paperwork, and it was emotionally hard dealing with the photos and the expert reports. I
needed to have the necessary forensic detail that would show what
happened. I remember spending time with the accident reconstruction expert – who had the measurements and was preparing a
report – I spent a few evenings with a Corgi car on the kitchen
table trying to work out how the car could have flipped over and
landed as it did. Writing witness and impact statements, poring
over documents, picking up points and discrepancies – preparing
for everything that might be of importance. I never prepared
myself for actually having to give evidence in court or expected it
to be a problem, as I knew the information inside out.

Being in the witness box was traumatic. I was exhausted and I
froze. I was repeatedly asked in a mocking tone to read my witness
statement. I kept trying to read it, but nothing went in. My brain
would not work. I was really embarrassed and felt humiliated. Not
my finest hour. Luckily it did not matter – the judge could see
what was happening and the witness statement was clear, so he just
allowed that in as evidence. Afterwards I went out into the corridor
and the barrister for the defence walked past me and said that I was
obviously lying as I could not remember my own story. I wanted to
go after him and walk into his office and state I was not lying – I
was stressed and overwhelmed. I thought about everything we had
been through, what had happened to Henry and our family, and his
life was ruined. I was absolutely enraged – I was not lying but I knew
they were lying and had tried to destroy records relating my brother's
accident. I was working in an area where I had access to these
documents and I obtained copies before they were destroyed by the
defendants. The judge made it very clear he was not impressed by
the defendants. He thought Henry was lucky to have his family.

The attitude of the judge echoed a theme that I became familiar with. My role in looking after Henry and supporting Mum defined me to others, as if I was doing something quite strange or remarkable. To me it was nothing like that, it was not good or bad, just necessary. This had happened and we had to give him the best quality of life we could – who else but us – we were his family. It was something that I had to do – and I needed to do it well. I don't know why I was the person that did it – I just was.

Mum and I had to take different roles with Henry. Mum was with him all the time, caring for him and helping him feel secure and keeping things calm. I dealt with anything that he would see as being confrontational, like finances, medical appointments and organising anything he had to do. I was very protective of him and felt great compassion but was also often irritated by his behaviour and had to suppress my responses – not always successfully!

When Henry loses his temper, he can be really 'in your face' – he can spit words out venomously and make hurtful, personal comments. After any of these tirades, it can sometimes leave me full of adrenalin, as I feel as if I have been attacked, and afterwards I feel mentally drained. I feel angry in the moment and then afterwards, sad and despondent. In the past I found it difficult to validate my own responses to his more challenging behaviour as I knew he couldn't help it because of his head injury. It seemed like I should know better than to feel that way, like being angry with a child for being overwhelmed. Mum and I are both aware that Henry cannot help much of his behaviour, because he has had a brain injury, but at odd moments, we still sometimes have to remind each other of this, if we are being wound up by him for any reason. Humour helps to diffuse situations.

I used to try and reason with him, but then realised he found it confronting and just made him angry, so it was pointless. He has a large 'ego', is always right and very rigid in his thinking and assumes people are talking about him.

There were attempts to help him be independent and attempts to set him up with carers, but these were all disasters and very stressful. By far the best solution and happiest for him was for mum to care for him. The search for and purchase of a suitable property took a long time and a lot of effort, but this was successful. Mum has given him so much and done an amazing job. I have so much admiration for her resilience and generosity.

Over time, I have become more of aware of how many of my stresses are related to events that have occurred and it has affected my health. I increasingly now have a 'what now?' response for any problems that come up – for any tasks that require concentrated effort.

Box 6.3 Professional reflection: ambiguous loss

In the telephone call, when Grace was describing her brother before the accident, she suddenly became tearful. She went on to say she had just had a visual image of her brother prior to the accident, when he was 'handsome', 'charming', 'laughing' and 'being silly', and she added, 'He died. The current Henry is different. It is such a waste'.

In a conversation with Grace the following day to confirm how she was, she said the discussion had been of value to her. She had thought about Henry, and reconnected to him as her brother, and was again more appreciative of the position he was stuck in. I was left with the feeling that it would have been worthwhile if I had initiated that conversation earlier.

Now I often procrastinate and then I feel guilty. The responsibility is always there, in the back of my head, placing pressure on me and guiding my decisions. I know the stuff will not go away but there are times I don't want to do it. I will then suddenly make up my mind to do it – and I do it quickly and sort it out.

Now, as I look back and consider everything, I recognise that, although I made choices as I went along, I do not really believe I had a choice. I made a decision to try and walk away and have a different life for a while after I had my children, but it did not work. I have never been able to achieve that, however much I may have wanted to at times. That is still the case.

I sometimes resented that I could not spend more time just with my mum. It was difficult for her to get away as she could not leave Henry. Mum and I are in it together – 'Partners in Enterprise'. I have a very strong, powerful bond with mum and that has increased as we have had so many intense emotional experiences together. We have been through so much together and been such a support for each other. Only someone else who has been on the same journey as us would understand.

I talk to her on the telephone every day to keep in touch and see how she is. There is shorthand communication between Mum and I. She can say what she wants to say, we banter. Mum and I laugh a lot and we hold each other together – we approach things through humour – that is how we operate. You may forget with whom you laughed, but you will never forget with whom you wept.

Henry is always there – there is nowhere to go to have a private conversation with mum at home, as he is always listening in and I get very irritated when he is occasionally indiscreet and discloses personal or inaccurate information about me or members of my family.

There are no solutions – just have to make the best of a bad situation. You cannot solve it – just get on with it.

Box 6.4 Professional reflections: meaning of life

In the interview Grace expressed the conflicts she had regarding coping with the situation, and during the interview she made the following statements:

> If someone came to me to ask me my view, I would want to say – do not do it – although morally I think they should. This is your family – who else's job is it? It is not easy to look after someone for a long length of time and never feel appreciated. He has no concept of what it costs others – he cannot appreciate or care. I sometimes find it hard to like him even though I know he can't help it – but then I often reflect that none of us would be show ourselves up to our great advantage if we had the brakes (social conditioning) removed.
>
> I love my brother and want to support him, even if this is challenging at times. I morally feel this is the right thing to do. I will always look after him and ensure that he has the best care and quality of life and organise whatever is required.
>
> One of the difficulties about being with him is him flipping between being unpleasant and being intensely vulnerable. One minute you want to strangle him and the next your heart is wrung. When he is being obsequious, that is stressful. There are still times when Henry can be hilarious – he makes mum and I laugh. He still has positive aspects of his original character, but he is also very different. I dread the time when Mum is not there.
>
> I am at peace with what I have done for Henry and do not regret it. I would do the same again if faced with the same situation – my regret is that at that time, I did not realise the impact on me or Mum and how it would affect us in the future.
>
> Would Henry have been better off if he had died? He does not seem to have a sense of gratitude for survival – or much insight into his

situation. There must be some purpose to his life and reasons why we have spent so much of our lives caring for him. For us, it is to do with Henry's quality of life; we do not want him to be in an institution because that is something that he fears. I sometimes wonder about wider impacts on the family.

The situation has curtailed our personal life, career prospects and income. I wanted to be there to support Mum and Henry. I am very fortunate, as my partner is massively supportive of me, Henry and my family. He finds it hard keeping still and quiet when Henry is shouting at me, my mum or my children. My partner wants to remove him from them, or vice versa. I stand up to Henry, but my mum and children do not fight back. My partner understands the fact that Mum and I support each other and, whenever there is a problem, he helps them. He does emergency dashes to the house whenever anything goes wrong, as Henry then becomes very agitated. This creates a stressful situation which needs resolving as soon as possible, and nobody else can get access because of Henry's condition. This reduces my stress levels and those of Mum and Henry. He wants to help Mum have an easier life. I am always aware of the need to safeguard my children from the challenges that arise with Henry. I do not lose sight of the need for them to have a normal childhood as far as possible, but this has not been easy when Henry has lost his temper suddenly and for no apparent reason.

I feel fortunate because after the court case we have had continuity of support from an experienced professional who has been with us for over 20 years. This often took pressure off me and also gave me valuable support at critical times. We would not have found it very easy or very helpful if we had had different people over this time, because establishing trust with new people would have been challenging for Henry, my mother and I.

Grace was asked if she had any messages for other siblings, and made the following suggestions:

- Seek out information early on.
- Consider the long-term effects of stress and the importance of your health to keep on doing the job that you are doing. Don't get run

down and get to the point of no return. Recognise and understand the stresses, make time for yourself and find something that nurtures you, so you can be there for the long term.

- Listen to the need behind the behaviour and what is actually going on, to see how to improve the situation.
- Learn to support them in the way they want, rather than in a way that you might think they need.
- Keep friends, have a social network and have things to refresh you. Keep your own life alive. Have boundaries and hold onto them. Don't let it define you.
- Try and keep sight of the relationship rather than the role.
- Try not to have too many people involved in making decisions for the care, but have a lot of support for the carers.
- The head injured are immensely difficult at times, but be kind. You will like yourself and them better if you can be.

Chapter 7

Children's challenges

As a case manager, I have worked with many clients with brain injury, who have had children of various ages. Some clients have children after the brain injury, so their offspring only know them as they are, whereas other children suffer the trauma of their parent's accident and recognise changes that have occurred.

Trauma affects a child's security, for instance, if both parents are missing and the child does not understand what has happened, and has to stay with extended family members or friends. Visiting a parent in hospital can be traumatic. At home, fatigue, unpredictable responses, loss of temper, or reduced abilities in everyday activities, are difficult to make sense of.

The type of input and support depends on the age of the child, their understanding of the situation, level of emotional distress and their ability to express concerns and communicate wishes. Over time, as children become older and when they are ready, support can be invaluable to help them make sense of what has occurred and enable them appreciate the alterations of the family roles and dynamics, and to find their own way forward.

Alistair, Beatrix and Christine

The first story is of two children (brother, Alistair, and sister, Beatrix), whose father sustained a brain injury when they were very young. They all lived together as a family and, although their father managed to work for a short time after the accident, he had to take medical retirement. The children wrote down their views of their childhood and the current situation, and Christine, their mother also provided comments to highlight her perspective of the family functioning. Alistair and Beatrix are now in their late 20s/early 30s; one of them is married with two young children, and the other child still lives at home.

Alistair and Beatrix reported on their father before the accident:

ALISTAIR: I was only 6 when his accident happened and although I have some memories of my early childhood, it's difficult to distinguish if they are from before or after. In reality, my dad has had a brain injury the entirety of my life.

BEATRIX: I'm told he had a great sense of humour, was very kind and compassionate – some of these qualities are still present, but he's not the same person. A piece of him died that day. I was recently looking through old photographs and comparing photos of Dad before and after the accident, you can see the difference in his face, behind his eyes the light is not there anymore, just a cold stare.

There were different perspectives of the accident

ALISTAIR: I recall the day of my dad's accident like it was yesterday and the choices that were made that could have resulted in a very different life. I vividly recall the first time I saw my dad in hospital following his accident. He was in a wheelchair and unable to speak. He was a shell of the man I called my dad. I had a new toy that was made of a slimy rubber material. He had a feel of it and turned up his nose. That was all he could do. I fought so hard to keep tears at bay as even at that age I knew that seeing me crying wasn't what he needed to see. Even to this day, it still brings tears to my eyes.

BEATRIX: Having been only two and a half when my dad sustained his head injury, I do not have the early memories that my brother has; my brother remembers that day vividly. I don't remember visiting him in hospital, or him coming home, or how he was before.

Alistair and Beatrix reflected on their childhood, on his behaviour consequent to his brain injury and how it impacted on their lives.

ALISTAIR: One minute he's Dr Jekyll – next he's Mr Hyde – Nearly every piece of kitchen crockery being smashed on the kitchen floor – Not going with him to his allotment the day he discovered his shed had been stolen and it being my fault. He's always tried to do dad stuff, like being supportive with sports and teaching DIY, but his approach hasn't been what it perhaps should have been. It's hard to say what impact my dads' brain injury has had on my life. To try and describe the impact I would really need an example of what would be considered 'normal' – to me, this has been normal.

I'm certain that it is not normal for most families, but it's the life I've lived. Having spent time in the company of other families, it's been far from normal in the extreme but there are others who have faced much worse in their upbringing.

BEATRIX: The impact on our family can only be described as shattering. We have been through a lot as a family, physical and mental abuse. Most of my childhood memories, unfortunately, are heavily loaded with abuse and fear of him. As a child/teenager, I remember spending a lot of time hiding in the bathroom behind a locked door and having to hold the lock, so he couldn't open it from the outside. He would not be satisfied or calm down until he got hold of you, for whatever you were meant to have done.

Our childhood was very different. His condition impacted us every day. Living with someone with a head injury is hard, very hard. The mood can change in a split second, or as we referred to it 'a flick of the light switch'. We have a saying in our household – he can be laughing with you and punch you in the face at the same time – the switch of moods can be so quick. We had to learn the signs of the mood changing, triggers that would set him off, and avoid them as much as possible or be prepared, if unavoidable. When he went back to work, you could tell the sort of evening it would be by the way he walked down the street. If he was marching, me and my brother prepared to go upstairs, if he slammed the gate, we were straight upstairs out the way. It doesn't take much for him to lose it – he doesn't have coping strategies; if a plan changes or something is not where it's meant to be, or someone hasn't/ isn't doing what he wants, we have a full-on meltdown – almost toddler tantrum style.

We had to do lots of things to help Dad, he would get very frustrated with himself if he couldn't fix something or do something, something that would have been second nature before the accident. We became very adept at holding the torch in the right place, getting the right screwdriver, holding things flush, we had little choice in the matter. Things have to be done his way. I do recall a fear of doing anything wrong or breaking anything as it was certain to set him off. In reality, it wasn't on purpose and no one was hurt, it happens. But he never could comprehend that.

Alistair and Beatrix both discussed the impact this had on the family unit and how they had all worked together to protect each other and taken on responsibilities that would not normally have been required for children of their age.

ALISTAIR: I guess in general, having to be a grown-up from an early age and protector of my mum and sister. In more recent years it's changed to being the rational one when my dad has worked himself up over something.

BEATRIX: Our roles over the years changed; Mum was mine and my brother's protector in the early years and she did her very best to shield us from him. Alistair was always very protective of me and took the brunt of the abuse when I was very young as a result. As me and my brother got older it would be us standing in front of Mum protecting her. It took for myself and Alistair to hit back as teenagers for him to realise he couldn't take out every anger or frustration on us – that we would fight back and were big enough and strong enough to stop him hurting us or Mum. Though he would still try. Violence shouldn't be used to stop violence, but this was the only method he understood, and it would only take us to push him back for him to realise it couldn't carry on. It is like living with a child, me as an adult now our roles are reversing even more, so I'm relied on heavily to deal with him.

Mine and my brother's relationship has always been very strong, we learnt very quickly that we needed to protect each other and continue to do so. We will always look out for each other and go above and beyond to help one another. We were each other's sole support as kids and could only talk to each other about it.

In 2006, my mum became seriously ill. As usual Dad showed very little concern for her and kept shouting for her to get up and tidy the house – same old story. I took her to the hospital, as he said he could not take her as he had an allotment meeting. A specialist told me my mother was very sick and asked whether I was next of kin. I called Dad to tell him, in no uncertain terms, to get his backside to the hospital. I'm 19 and terrified that Mum is dying in front of me. He got restless waiting for Mum to be moved to ICU in the hospital, so I asked him to take one of the cars home, so he had something to do and this needed to be done. He then had a shower and spent ages at home looking for his radio Walkman! Why? Because the World Cup was on and England were playing that afternoon. He needed it so he could listen to the match! A surgeon is trying to put a central line in mum and he's trying to find out what station the football is on. The moment of realisation for him that he could lose his wife is when Mum has to go for a CT of her kidneys and the doctors, nurses and porter are arguing where to put the 'big red bag'. Once they decide, he asks me 'What is the big red bag for?' I tell him it's a resuscitation pack, with a portable defibrillator and drugs to resuscitate Mum should she crash. He looks at the nurse to confirm what I just said and then the look on his face changes, the realisation that she could die and that he would be left on his own dawns on him.

CHRISTINE: I had to take on both roles – mum and dad. Be the protector/argue on the children's behalf /negotiator. In 2006 when I was in hospital his attitude was anger towards the children – however, his behaviour improved somewhat as he knew he would have been on his own if I had died – as the children were old enough to fend for themselves. Alistair has always been protective of Beatrix since the accident. Alistair, being older, and along with me, was always blamed for lots of things and often punished. As he got older he defended himself and us. They're always protective of me when he does public rants and they also won't take any stick from others either – they stand up for their rights!

Beatrix talked about their relationships with her father's parents.

BEATRIX: His relationships with his family always seemed strange to me, they weren't very caring towards him and did very little to help us. They were very blasé about the abuse he inflicted on us. Now following some family revelations, we kind of understand why they were so strange. He had a very strained relationship with his father, which wasn't helped by me and my brother adoring him. It hurt Dad to see us playing with Granddad, him teaching us how to play badminton and taking us swimming and over the park – and he could run after us whereas Dad struggled.

Alistair and Beatrix both talked about how it affected them when they were with their father and met people, including their own friends.

ALISTAIR: It's always been awkward to explain that my dad has had a brain injury to new people who meet him. I don't think they've fully understood what that means and in all honesty, it's difficult to explain.

BEATRIX: He has no people-skills, doesn't know when to shut up, says inappropriate things and upsets people; this makes it difficult to introduce him to new people. You've half scared them off when you are briefing them on what he's like.

ALISTAIR: Had a cricket match at school which Dad came to watch. As he was limping across the field, one of the guys in my year said 'Who's that weirdo?' Errr, that's my dad.

BEATRIX: Relationships with some friends were hard, some close friends would not invite us as a family to their events as, as they put it 'we would have to ask him'. This was very hard to hear when I was younger, because to me I knew no different – he was my dad – and he was being treated differently because he had a head injury. He was excluded from a lot of things because of his head injury, which meant we were too. Some people just couldn't handle how he is. The thing they don't understand is when he is out in public or around someone else's house he is on his best behaviour and tries his best to be as normal as possible.

Alistair and Beatrix highlighted their perspectives of having a lost childhood.

ALISTAIR: It's now that I'm married and have my own child, I realise that there are a lot of things I've missed when growing up. Family days out to the zoo etc., and family holidays abroad. To the point I now find these things difficult to enjoy and appreciate, as I've never experienced them before and don't know what to expect.

BEATRIX: We missed out as kids going to theme parks and on holidays, because of his condition. I don't think he has ever been to a theme park in his life, and we couldn't have risked it in the early years, have him kick off in the middle of a theme park – he would have probably wound up arrested.

When reflecting on their childhood, Alistair and Beatrix highlighted the lack of understanding of brain injury and attitudes of others.

BEATRIX: We were not prepared for what we were going to live with; it seemed to me that, after a couple of years, the hospital kind of wiped their hands of him and left us to it. It was more difficult back then to tell us what it would be like. It seemed like head injuries were a taboo subject. People that met Dad did think he had a mental illness.

People don't understand people with head injury – they don't understand that it takes them a very long time to process anything – they don't handle stress or change. They need to ask lots of questions – this can be really frustrating for you and them. They may ask the same question in five different ways and the answer be the same, but this is how they are trying to understand and process it. You have to keep to the facts and precise answers, no maybes and exact times, 4 p.m.-ish does not work. It takes a great deal of patience to live with.

ALISTAIR: Back in the 90s and early 00s it was hard to be disabled, especially with a head injury. You were looked at differently and definitely treated differently. Now in 2018 everyone is very PC about disability and it's much more accepted. In the beginning he didn't want to be referred to as disabled, he didn't want to be a disabled man. Now he won't shut up about it: rights for disabled people, telling shop owners off if their door is not wide enough to fit a wheelchair, someone parking in a disabled parking spot without a badge, to name a few.

Alistair and Beatrix were asked what had positively made a difference to their lives or helped them over time.

ALISTAIR: Not sure there is anything that has really made a difference, and day to day, nothing springs to mind. We've had to get on and do the best we can.

BEATRIX: Time and acceptance. Over the years he has mellowed, in comparison to what he was like. It's still like living with Jekyll and Hyde though. It took a long time for him to accept that he wasn't going to be like he was before. He was very envious of my brother and I think resented him. He could see in my brother the man he was, my brother could run, swim, play rugby, play cricket – all the things he had once done.

Alistair and Beatrix both highlighted the importance of friends to survive.

ALISTAIR: Having close family friends has helped. It was a great help to have close friends and family; however, I can only surmise it is like soldiers coming home from war: you're somewhere safe, away from the conflict, but it's not right, you feel awkward, you don't know how to act, it's not normal. I think that I have lost and continue to lose friends because I lack a level of comfort in situations.

BEATRIX: We would spend a lot of time across the road at our neighbours with their daughters. They became family to us, even to this day. They were there from day one – helped Mum on the day of his accident, our neighbour drove Mum to the hospital while he looked after me and my brother. They were our lifeline or safe place when Dad would start to turn: the only thing Mum could do to protect us was to get us out of sight, which would either be upstairs or across the street. Without our neighbours we would have not survived as children.

CHRISTINE: I removed them from the situation when possible – he can shout and hit you and then ten minutes later will treat you as if nothing has happened! Although they didn't always like being at their grandparents I did encourage holidays for them to be away from the home situation. Alistair would make us leave the house and go to grandparents' if things were really bad and also, at times, I phoned the case manager to help diffuse the situation.

Alistair and Beatrix reported on participating in enjoyable activities or hobbies that distracted them from the situation at home, and ideas for activities their father could do without them.

ALISTAIR: Probably having a hobby that pulls you away from the home environment and gives you independence from the situation has been the greatest help. A break from the tense environment.

BEATRIX: We coped a lot by being out of the house away from him; we used to do lots of things in the evenings without him. Both me and my brother swam for the local team, so that kept us busy several times a week on top of brownies/guides and cubs/scouts. The weekends and school holidays were the hardest. He never liked school holidays, even before his accident, because Mum was a teacher and so she got more time off than he did. This made it more difficult after his accident, and when we were both in school it got to the stage where we spent a large chunk of our holiday with Mum's family and away from him. We began to lead a separate life from him.

BEATRIX: Someone suggested to him about getting an allotment to pass his time, which helped. He could be over there for most of the day some days.

Alistair and Beatrix described the value of the case management input to them during their childhood.

ALISTAIR: Having the support of a case management company, our case manager has always been a phone call away.

BEATRIX: Our lifeline was our case manager. Having a 'phone a friend' as it were, was beneficial to us. She could spend hours talking to him, to find out what the problem was that made him kick off and help him resolve that issue. He would be a different person when he came off the phone. Hers was a number we each had written in multiple places for easy access to call to get her to help. The case manager saved us from a beating on far too many an occasion. I was told that we were a family that if we, or someone for us, called the case management office and the person thought we were in serious danger, they had permission and the phone number to call our local police station to get us help. Says a lot about what we lived with.

Box 7.1 Professional reflection: need for safety and immediate support

I recall these telephone conversations as if they were yesterday. They did not occur very often but, at that time, I was always on call and alert to all issues that could arise. If I was away, other case managers were alert to the needs of this family and would have taken the same approach. Calls to the children were often brief, as they were reporting in, but I always confirmed they were safe prior to ringing their father back to talk through the issues that were causing his temper outburst. They and I knew that I (and others) could reduce his levels of agitation and anger by talking through the issues with him, and by being on the telephone with him we would also remove him from the direct confrontations or frictions that were occurring in the family unit. Their father never knew the children rang. He never worked out the coincidence of the timing of calls to him, i.e. that they occurred when he was having a temper tantrum.

These scenarios were a long time ago, before the current safeguarding regulations, so in our communication further information was sought from the children about their views about whether these incidents should have been reported to Social Services.

ALISTAIR: (who works in the police force): I'm certain that if what we went through was in today's society/climate, I'm not sure my sister and I would still be with our parents, certainly not my dad, as he was at the beginning.

BEATRIX: We were told as children not to tell anyone about Dad and what happened at home. It was always scared into us that if we told, Social Services would come and take me and my brother away. None of our teachers were told; they only discovered when I was choosing my GCSEs and he had to come to parents' evening. We hid our lives and our bruises. I was asked by a teacher why we hadn't informed school what we lived with at home, as allowances could have been made for me and my brother, and my answer was why do we need allowances? Aren't we performing well enough in school? Why do we need special treatment? We have been living with this since 1989. This surprised my teacher greatly. She said I was too mature for my age. Me and my brother always lived with the philosophy 'what doesn't kill us makes us stronger'.

I think we would have benefited from being monitored. Both me and my brother wouldn't have wanted to be treated differently in school, but having teachers aware would have made school life easier for us. Just having them understand what we lived with at home and realising why some days we were in school ridiculously early, and just having a teacher see something was wrong and giving us support in school. We needed the support that comes with social services; the only support we really had was from the case management company and some from the hospital in the beginning.

Box 7.2 Professional reflection: safeguarding

I remember struggling with the safeguarding issue at this time, on how and when to report to Social Services, and what they would do. The consequences of brain injury were not well recognised at this time and, whilst trying to support their father on developing strategies to reduce his agitation and aggression, he had limited insight (i.e. he did not recognise he had any problems) and would not accept any neuropsychological interventions. He did not progress.

I was very concerned about the situation and the children's well-being and discussed this with Christine frequently. Christine fluctuated in her views about whether she was going to leave her husband or not. She felt guilty about the idea of leaving him, as he could not cope alone, whilst also trying to protect her children.

I knew that if I reported to Social Services, at that time, Christine would sack me (which she confirmed she would have done in a recent telephone call) and then the children would not have support available to them, as and when required.

I talked the issue through with a social worker I worked with, and I know she reported to Social Services, who investigated but did not do anything. Christine was furious about this report to Social Services, as they visited her at home and saw the children at school. She felt they had criticised her parenting rather than highlighting the issue of how to support her in managing her husband's behaviour towards the children.

Alistair, Beatrix and Christine, were asked for their perspective on what could have happened if they had not stayed together as a family.

BEATRIX: Whatever he says, he would not have survived without us looking after him. He would have been abandoned if we left, his family would not have looked after him, he would have either ended up on the streets or dying.

CHRISTINE: If this accident were to happen again and we were faced with the option of turning off the life support – I would not hesitate. I'll never know if I did the right thing staying with him – but then again, I come across so many kids from broken homes and I didn't want to be classed as one of them. Alistair did say to me last year, 'do you mean that bloke you should have divorced 20 years ago?' – I didn't know he felt like that. If a social worker had removed the kids, I would have gone with them. The thing is the only place I would have wanted to go to was home to my mum – and that wouldn't have been fair to the kids as I would have no hope of getting a job there – financially they would have lost out. If she had lived closer, I would have left. He is kind to us all in different ways – depending on his mood – but the bad ones outweigh the good unfortunately! On a bad day I think I should have left, and on other days I cope. We'll continue to plod on!

ALISTAIR: My wife recently asked me that if I could go back and change it, would I stop my dad going to work that day? But in answer to the question: No. I wouldn't change it. I may have had a difficult upbringing and, sometimes, a violent existence. There may have been a large amount of love lost and a stolen childhood, but I am the person I am today because of it. I like to think that I've turned out alright, although I'm sure I have my faults. We've remained a family (I'm not quite sure how) throughout and who's to say that if he hadn't had his head injury that would be the case?

BEATRIX: It's difficult to say if a more normal upbringing would have been better; to us as kids it was normal, we knew no different. Yes, we should have been more protected from him and no, because it made us the people we are today, we are stronger for it.

We were one of the only families to have stayed together – madness really when you think about it, what we put up with for all these years and still put up with. Think we could do with some serious therapy.

If it was me (instead of Mum) in the same situation, I would leave and move away with my kids and only allow supervised visits. I wouldn't be able to put myself through that again and definitely not my kids, no child should go through what me and my brother went through and witnessed.

If we had left Dad, the only place Mum would have gone was back to her home area [about 200 miles away from where they lived]. This would have been difficult. My brother was in school and Mum would have struggled to get a job, and we would have struggled with money. It would also have made it much harder to see Dad. Weekend visits would have been a nightmare – he would have worked himself up – they would have needed to be supervised – and Mum definitely kept away from him. I remember very clearly the time we ran from him and went to my grandparents. On our return to the house and him, the case manager met us at the end of the road to mediate the exchange of us coming home. We would have needed a mediator at every interaction.

Alistair and Beatrix were asked about whether there were concerns they had now, in respect of their father, for the future.

ALISTAIR: I think the biggest thing that scares me is to turn out like my dad. Not in the sense of having a brain injury, but to be like him towards my own wife and children. It's the example that was set to me and I don't wish to default to that.

BEATRIX: It's sad now that with my brother's children, it's a rule between me and him that the kids are never left alone with Dad. There always has to be either me, my brother or his wife in the room. We can't trust him with his own grandsons. We couldn't risk him smacking them if they did something wrong. He doesn't look after them or protect them. He wouldn't be able to soothe them if they fell over and hurt themselves for example. He has no social awareness and they would pick up bad habits and inappropriate things. It's sad that we have to limit the interaction with them, but he can't handle it. Alistair's son loves his granddad, but Dad gets ratty quickly or will start an argument with Mum, which we don't want the kids to have to deal with.

BEATRIX: He will get the hump if we arrange a family event when there is something on TV he wants to watch; for example, take Alistair's son's first birthday party, we ended up having to leave early because he wanted to go home. He and my brother had had words, as Dad wanted to watch the Grand Prix instead of being at the party. It really upset my brother that he would rather be watching the TV than participate in his grandson's birthday. Which meant me and Mum missed out. We had to take him home, as I drove. We are getting to the stage where he's not invited anymore, as it's easier.

Alistair and Beatrix were asked whether they had any messages for other children in this position.

ALISTAIR: The injury may have had a significant impact on your life and it will shape your life for years to come, but it doesn't have to be your life. Yes, you live with the consequences and the hardships, but let it shape you for the better. Enjoy the good times, weather the storm that are the bad times and do something that is solely for you, so you have that separation.

BEATRIX: Be patient, be strong, be brave and have support. If I knew then what I know now, my life could have been different. I wish I had fought back earlier, and protected myself more. If they are violent, they will always say they are sorry, they didn't mean it and they couldn't help it. Yes, they are sorry, they do regret their actions and they will get very upset when it sinks in what they just did. And yes, in that moment, they did mean it. Their brain hasn't processed what they are doing is wrong and this is their only way out. And yes, they can help it. They just need to want to, they need to want to work on themselves and think their actions through. Hitting someone will not solve their problem.

Have people to support you, whether it is friends, family, neighbours or a support group. You will need help, you will need time away and need to talk to someone. Don't be scared to ask for help, friends that treat you differently because of the head injury are not your friends and you don't need them in your life.

And if you can't cope, don't feel guilty for walking away, it may be the best thing for you and them.

Box 7.3 Professional reflection: discrepancies

I value the open and honest opinions expressed by Alistair, Beatrix and Christine in respect of their situation, especially considering how this continues to impact on their day-to-day lives. There has been little change in their father since his brain injury. He acknowledges his physical deficits but lacks insight in the effects of his brain injury and the impact of his behaviour and lack of empathy on those around him, including his family.

I was involved in working with this family for about ten years, up until the time the children became older and strong enough to stand up and challenge their father. Whilst I could discuss issues with their father, so he could appreciate alternative viewpoints and ways to handle situations in the moment, it did not change his behaviour over time. He would default to his fixed, stereotyped ways of thinking and make demands on others to dance to his tune, in all aspects of his home and community life.

Different members of the family have different views about what decisions they think they would have made or what they would have liked to have seen happening. It is all so difficult in reality. As in so many everyday situations, there is no real answer as to what can be deemed to be right, or how it could have been if different decisions had been made. This family have survived, but at what cost?

Deidre

The second story is that of 'child' Deidre, who was in her early thirties when both of her parents were involved in a road traffic accident. Her mother died, and her father sustained a severe brain injury. Deidre's father resided in a nursing home and had additional one-to-one care from support workers that Deidre employed. During the interview with Deidre, her father was in his 80s and deteriorating; there was discussion about his end of life care. The poignancy of knowing Deidre throughout the time from shortly after his accident to his demise was reflected in the conversation. Deidre's father died whilst this chapter was being written.

Deidre talked in detail about the accident, about what occurred before and immediately afterwards. She said,

> It had been a bizarre week – my parents had been staying with me – they picked me up from work, as I had a problem with my car. All week, every time I was in the car, I was convinced something was going to hit them. The last memory of my parents was of them in bed before I went to work, and they left to return home. I remember Viscount Linley got married at the time of my parent's accident.
>
> I have a playback of what happened on the day of the accident – I worked that day and, in the evening, was babysitting my godson and staying the night.

Deidre recalled everything in fine detail. As Deidre was not at home, people had difficulty contacting her to inform her of her parents' accident, and after receiving the call she did not know what to do, as she could not leave her godson alone. Deidre tried to contact her friends, via the school where they were, to ask them to come back, and then she had difficulty communicating with her family so she could find out which hospital to go to. Deidre said the police were looking for her after the incident but could not find her.

Deidre shared her recollections from the hospital.

> I was given the Help the Aged leaflet on bereavement in ICU, as mum had been killed, as that was all they had.
>
> On the ward, they were not used to people with brain injury and my dad used to take things and wander off with them. They blamed him when anything went missing.
>
> My dad had to see a psychiatrist, as he was agitated, and at that time I went along with what professionals suggested. The psychiatrist prescribed him a massive dose of chlorpromazine. I have an image of my dad standing with an apron on at the nurses' station; he was pill rolling in less than a week due to the excessive dose of medication and he has had a Parkinsonian tremor ever since.
>
> I lived in Oxford at that time, so Dad came to Oxford for his rehabilitation. I was working full-time or visiting Dad. There was no opportunity for a life in between. My brothers could not visit my father very often in Oxford, as they were married and had young children – so it was down to me.
>
> After the accident I even had to teach him how to go the toilet again and manage his bowels – I wanted to help him do what he could.

Deidre said that the worst experience she had was when her father was in a rehabilitation unit and the nurse in charge rang her when she was working and formally told her that, if her father got out again (he was known to wander), they would not be following him.

> I was beside myself and had to take two days compassionate leave from work to see what could be done. It transpired that the rehabilitation unit had found a care facility (a distance away) and arranged for him to be moved, without any communication with me, as they wanted him away from their unit.

Deidre and one of her brothers collected her father from this rehabilitation unit and took him to a care facility.

Deidre had issues with work, as she was ill and had to take time off sick, but her employers thought she was not managing her work. Deidre felt they did not treat her sympathetically considering the circumstances she was dealing with.

I moved back to the area that I grew up in, as living in Oxford was 'unsustainable' and I felt it was right for my father to come back to this area. My brothers lived there. Coming back was really difficult. Then I was working full-time, visiting him every weekend, and he often stayed overnight at weekends in my home.

Deidre described the impact of the accident and her father's brain injury on her life.

At the time of the accident my mum was 52. Mum and I were very close. I knew if this happened to my mother, she would not want to be in a care home, as my dad has been, but I could not manage it any other way. My grandmother died the same year as my mother. Now I am older than my mum when she was killed.

I was 31, single and I hoped to marry and have a family. The accident and everything associated with it changed that course for me. It impacted on my opportunities and I was not emotionally available to do anything other than care for my father and be there for the family. It took me until about five years after the accident before I could start developing new social networks. I have had a relationship now for the past 10 to 12 years but he knows I have a strong attachment with my dad and his needs are paramount.

After the accident suddenly I was the grown up – parent to my father overnight – my father was 58. I have never had children, but I feel a maternal feeling towards my father. I feel the need to be there. I am the lioness, who will do anything to protect my dad and ensure he has whatever he needs and is cared for to the standard he should be cared for.

I feel as if I have been on an emotional rollercoaster – I felt guilt for years after the accident, as at times I wished he had died. Five years after the accident, I had a party here in my house and my father was sitting on a chair. He looked just like my dad before the accident. I remember thinking, you can wake up and be my dad again now. I was robbed of my dad – he was gone in an instant. Knowing all the things I know now – relatives do not know how it can happen. I thought the worst thing that could have happened was if my parents had both died, but that is not true, the worst situation would have been if they had both sustained a head injury.

I am a nurse – at the time of the accident I was a midwifery sister – and I know the health systems and have access to those systems, and I know the right things to say and the right words to use. I felt this is what I had done my training for. I have had to compartmentalise my home and work life. I have covered my father's personal care sometimes, and covered shifts at the home as required, but I am mindful that I am his daughter, not his nurse. However, I have also had to approach the staff on the unit, as a nurse, when aspects of his care have needed to be addressed.

Dad is constantly agitated, has no short-term memory and cannot make any sense of the world. He cannot articulate what he wants, like asking for a drink, or have a conversation, and has not been able to do that for 25 years. I ring my dad at the same time every night and my dad says, is that Deidre? Christmases have always been centred around my dad. I took him home overnight when he was fit enough for this, but then he just came for the day. He could not do this last year, as he was too ill and tired. When my dad returned home for Easter or Christmas, it was very hard, as I was up during the night to change him and then had to put him back to bed. One time I made Sunday lunch for 13 people and my dad had no awareness of danger, and on one occasion he went to put his hand into the hot tin of roast potatoes. My dad repeats statements and phrases constantly, as he cannot remember he has already said them. On one occasion, when I was doing some ironing and he wanted to sit on a different chair, which would have involved moving the ironing board, he made the same comment to me 20 times in 15 minutes. Even though I asked him if he could wait, he forgot and eventually, I had to move the ironing board to allow this to occur.

I still feel guilt when wishing him dead – he is only just about there – physically – not really awake very often. Now he is sometimes bright – he smiles when he sees me – other than that – not a lot back. For half my life I have been responsible for my dad and I have forgotten what life was like before the accident. I have had stress all the time, even when on holiday, and I worry about saying 'goodbye'.

Deidre shared her perspective of the impact of the accident and her father's brain injury on the family.

I took over the role of being the key person to communicate and try to keep the family together.

The accident affected my brothers. One of my brothers had a divorce and he said he felt he had to live life at 100 miles an hour to make the most of it.

I do not think it has changed my relationship with my brothers – they might think I took over. One brother has always said I should have a life, not forget my own life, and tells me that I spend too much time with Dad. It has not harmed our relationship – he has tried to protect me.

My brothers find it difficult to visit him and see Dad as he is. He has no social communication. He only remembers my name. I have constantly told my family that Dad was pleased to see them and that he knows who they are, but he cannot necessarily say their names. I cannot predict how my dad will be or when will be the right time for family to visit him.

Deidre described relationships with friends.

I find it difficult sometimes, as my friends have parents the same age as my father and they are expressing how their parents are becoming more dependent on them. I have been doing this since the age of 31, whereas they are only having this experience now.

Deidre was asked what she had found helped her over the past 25 years, and she said she felt reassured by the fact that her father had the care he needed.

I have taken great comfort from the fact that someone is with my dad and that he has the level of care we want him to have. From his court settlement we paid for my dad to have one-to-one carers and they know him well. I have a good laugh with these girls and they have good knowledge about my father and how he likes everything to be done. For instance, Dad is funny about the way he takes his jumper off. I am so lucky to have carers so loyal to him.

In my experience staff at the care home lack understanding of brain injury and, if they do not know my father well, it can create problems, as he does not initiate anything. For instance, staff will place a glass by the side of my dad and leave it there. He needs prompting to drink. Staff will pin a bell to him, but he would never think about pressing it.

Deidre discussed the litigation process, which provided the finance to pay for his care.

> Money brings power. My dad had a structured settlement and that has kept the wolf from the door to allow for Dad to have the care he has needed. If that had not been possible, I would have given up work and cared for Dad at home. That would have been to the detriment of my health and would have been very hard on our relationship.
>
> One of my brothers was initially more involved in the court case but somehow, because I was single and a nurse, the majority of it fell to me. There was extreme pressure when trying to deal with litigation, as I was training to be a health visitor, working as a nurse and supporting my father. I had little free time. I prepared witness statements and had to take my father to see the experts. My brothers would always go with me and Dad if they were asked to. I felt they [the experts] were trying to trip me up the whole time. I remember the experts would say he was going to die and not need so much money. He lived far longer than they said he would.

Deidre talked about how difficult it was to establish the support she needed.

> I have a friend whose sibling had a brain injury on the same day as my father and we have shared experiences and that has been mutually supportive.
>
> I was a square peg in a round hole. I was 31, not a child and not a parent, and I do not feel anything really worked for me. I chaired and ran a Headway group for a time, but withdrew, as that did not help. I felt I was always there and supporting other people. I have not joined in with the relatives' meetings at the nursing home, partly because I am a nurse. I have never fitted with anything as I have not had the same shared experiences.
>
> I have colleagues with skills. If I do not know what to do, I know someone that does. I talked to a Mental Capacity Lead before I organised an end of life plan for my father – she helped me frame my conversation with the GP.

Deidre described fears she has developed since the accident and how she manages these.

> I always like people to know where I am and where other people are, in the event of anyone being needed.

I go horse riding and am constantly afraid that by doing any of the things I do, that I could have a brain injury like my dad.

I worry about being on holiday and something happening to my father. I did not say goodbye to my mum.

I worry about people who do not have the knowledge that I have, as they do not know who to go to or how the system works.

Deidre was asked what messages she could give to others, if they were in this situation.

One thing I have said to people in these situations: make decisions, and at the end of the day when judgement day comes, and it is all over, you can be perfectly at peace with what you have done. Do not wish for or regret what you could have done.

I have to ask questions and learn. People need to keep asking and feel satisfied they have the right answer and, if not happy, to continue asking. Fundamentally we believe what is acceptable. If we do not believe it is right for us or our standards – it is not.

Knowledge is power. I have always felt that. If people lack confidence or are not well informed, it puts them at a disadvantage. I believe how you dress for an occasion gives you power. When I went to meetings smartly dressed and appeared confident, I felt on a level footing and was treated differently.

Box 7.4 Professional reflection: knowledge is power

Deidre's knowledge and experience has allowed her to be an excellent advocate on behalf of her father, for what she believed he needed and wanted.

Our case management involvement started when Deidre's father was confused and would wander off down the road from a care facility (which was situated in a remote location), sometimes in his pyjamas. He was unsupervised and highly at risk. We supported Deidre in establishing a consistent group of carers to work with her father, providing supervision, assistance and companionship in his everyday life. These carers worked with him for years and knew him well.

As a case manager, I provided a support system behind the scenes, as required, to support Deidre. The support was in situations where Deidre's emotional responses to inconsistent standards of care or poor professional practice caused her distress, and interventions were required with staff at the care facilities or statutory authorities to resolve the issues that arose.

Deidre was proactive to ensure everything was considered in advance, so her father could be provided with the best care possible. Her father's quality of life was significantly improved as a consequence of Deidre's committed concern for his health and welfare. She could not have done anything more and, when he died, she knew that. In communication with Deidre after her father's death, she commented that she was just 'going with the flow'.

Chapter 8

The impact of acquired brain injury on the family

Common themes, threads and differences

The beautifully scripted narratives in the previous chapters describe these relatives' reflections on how they have, and continue to, live with the consequences of brain injury. Everyone has their own story to tell, which is core to their 'way of being', and they express their values and beliefs of what is important to them, and to their relative with the brain injury. The relatives were all focused on being able to help others learn from their experiences; it is the reason why they agreed to contribute to this book.

In this chapter, the relatives' narratives are reviewed to identify the common threads and themes, and those which are unique to their personal experience, the relationships they have and the roles they fulfil. By doing so we hope to emphasise similarities and differences within the stories told. This will provide a greater level of understanding of the lived experiences of family members but will also point towards how to best provide support for individuals in similar situations.

Context before the accident

All the narratives provided the context, so we could gain greater understanding of the person who had sustained the trauma, within the context of their family and lifestyle. We can appreciate the injured individuals' values, prospects, ambitions, interests and relationships, whilst also being able to reflect these from the perspectives of the hopes and wishes of the relative who has told their story.

Jeanne and Dan described their respective sons, Adam and Paul, who at the time of their injuries were going through transitions, for instance achieving success in their education, working towards their careers and developing independent lives. They were enjoying their lives in a way that was utterly normal for that family. Jeanne's husband had a full-time executive job with a strong marriage and children, and all to live for. Deidre had been enjoying the company of her parents at her home just prior to the accident and had hopes to develop a relationship, marry and have children. Grace described an on-off relationship she had with her brother prior to the accident. Eliza described a normal sibling relationship, with a sister who was always rather headstrong and wilful and with very supportive parents. Alistair and Beatrix were really too young to remember their father before the accident or their own thoughts about the future.

Traumatic event and the immediate aftermath

The trauma

The traumas that occurred were all sudden and life-changing. In the narratives all the relatives, apart from the young children, could remember exactly where they were and what they were doing when they heard of their relatives' accident. They could relate all the fine detail with great clarity and in some cases relive the experience. These memories have not faded over time.

Some relatives were present immediately after the accident and traumatised by what they saw and heard. Jeanne could graphically relate the aftermath of the accident, even 23 years later. She heard about the incident from her daughter, observed her son lying on the ground, and she interacted with others and recalls the blood of his injured friends. Dan said, '*I remember the blood … but more the cut to his temple sticks in my mind. I remember praying he had not hurt his head, you just know if someone hurts their head it cannot be repaired.*' Laura provided in-depth information about finding her husband collapsed in the spare bedroom and trying to support her children, whilst also needing to be with her husband. Deidre heard about her parent's accident by telephone, when she was not in a position to leave the house as she was babysitting. She relived the panic she had at the time, in trying to get relevant information about her parents and communicate with friends to relieve her of her babysitting responsibilities. It was noticeable that the siblings and younger children did not recall any of these details in the interview.

There was a description of how fear changed their perception of time – '*probably only a few minutes but it felt like forever*' – when waiting for emergency interventions.

The relatives had to manage the immediacy of their crisis, for instance their existing responsibilities and commitments, the safety of children or dependents, and communication with relevant others who needed to immediately know about the accident. There was little else they could do.

Coping in the early stages

The members of the family commonly described being in '*a haze*' and '*waking up from a nightmare*' – '*waiting*' – their immediate uncertainties and background worries for their futures. Relatives relied on hope that everything would be ok and return to 'normal'.

Relatives were generally positive about the care of their injured relatives in the Intensive Care Unit, as they could be there and see the one-to-one commitment of the nurses working with their relative to support their survival and recovery. Jeanne described her bewilderment with all the machinery and bleeping noises.

Laura, Dan, Jeanne and Deidre needed to be with their injured sons/husband/father at the hospital, often staying overnight in the ICU. They needed to be there because of the uncertainty of whether their relative was going to survive or not, and going to emerge from coma, and if so when. News of their relative's condition led to emotional 'ups and downs' and extremes of views, i.e. from '*everything is going to be ok*' to '*they are going to die*'.

Dan feared what he did not know; if Paul was going to wake up, who he would be or what he would be like? He did not know how to deal with what was happening. He said it was a life changing moment when his son woke from coma and asked him who he was. Dan commented he was not functioning all that well in the weeks and months post injury, even though he thought he was. The passage of time has enabled him to review this.

Laura described her husband's move to the stroke ward. After the calm of the Intensive Care Unit, she had to cope with her husband in a 'dire' environment, where patients were coming and going, day and night, and she overheard doctors' conversations with other patients.

Jeanne's son fell out of bed shortly after being transferred to a general ward. The family had to provide care 24 hours a day (in hospital) to ensure his safety and the nursing staff welcomed their input. Jeanne said her son was very frightened, unable to make sense of the world and he was verbally, and sometimes physically aggressive. Adam thought the staff on the unit were trying to harm him, so they had to be with him whenever he was awake. When she was not present, he rang his mother at least 15 times a day.

The siblings and younger children visited their sibling/father in hospital. Whilst some of the older siblings were supporting their respective siblings, they were not taking primary responsibility, as that was the role of their parent(s). Alistair described his memory of the first time he saw his father in hospital after the accident and how, if he thinks about it, this still emotionally upsets him now, decades later.

Family members highlighted how overwhelming this initial experience in hospital was and focusing on anything other than their injured relative was very difficult. Relatives felt that remaining alert at all times was essential, in case they were required to be there for their relative. The family member needed to know what was happening at all times.

Laura highlighted how, in the initial stages, she had difficulty dealing with the conflicting needs of her injured partner and her children. They were all traumatised, but she could not be with them all at the same time. She described how she was always open and honest with the children, shared heart-breaking news and was led by their questions and needs, so they felt more reassured and were less afraid. Laura described feeling overwhelmed in trying to do everything, for instance juggling hospital visiting every day, taking and collecting the children from school and managing everything at home.

Laura described the trauma at a review meeting of her husband, when he was on the stroke ward. She felt she was being interrogated by a room full of doctors, therapists and nurses she hardly knew. They were all talking about their views of her husband's needs and potential discharge plans, before this had been discussed with her and she had no idea how she could cope with him at home. She was able to feed back her negative experience of this meeting to the ward sister.

Different family members talked about how other relatives and friends stepped in to look after their children, supported them and provided help when decisions needed to be made, and dealt with other practical issues. Laura felt positively about people who 'went out of their way' to help and support her.

On discharge home

The neuropsychologist thought it would be better for Adam to be discharged home, as he lacked awareness of his limitations. Jeanne and the family were left to care for Adam. At this time the family did not understand the deficits caused by Adam's brain injury, for instance poor memory, anger, changeable moods, disinhibition and lack of executive functioning. They did not receive any instruction as to what to do, nor any support or information.

Dan said Paul's condition did not make sense to him or the family. He just noticed Paul had unusual behaviours and had to be told what to do.

Grace said, '*it not did make any sense to us at the beginning*'.

Eliza commented on the strained and tense environment at her parents' home, due to the volatility of the sister's behaviour. Everybody had to dance to her tune to keep the peace.

Laura's husband, John, has remained in a slow stream rehabilitation setting in a bungalow with five other residents. Laura felt it was a positive space for the family to visit John as a family.

Longer-term ups and downs for family

All the relatives graphically expressed the issues that had arisen for them over long periods of time. The following themes emerged:

Duty and responsibilities over time

It was evident from the contributions that some family members assumed the role (or were assigned the role) of being the primary family member responsible for their injured relative. Dan saw his duty to stand up for his family values and support his injured son above anything else. He and Jeanne took on these responsibilities, supported by their partners, and Laura, as spouse, was next of kin for John. Deidre acknowledged that she was left to get on with it, as her siblings had commitments and did not know what to do, and she was single and an experienced nurse. All of these family members have maintained these responsibilities over very lengthy periods of time. Dan and Jeanne continue to do so, even though the circumstances have changed. Deidre took full responsibility for managing her father's care throughout his life and right up to his death.

Grace and her mother have shared the responsibilities for her brother. Grace's life changed when she had children, and she has taken one step back from the direct support of her brother but continues to do anything she can to support her brother and mother.

Eliza's parents took primary responsibility for her sister and it was only as her parents grew older that she provided backup support to them in the care of her sister. When they died, she took over this responsibility and continues to be there to this day.

Alistair and Beatrix have never taken primary responsibility for their father's care, although when her mother was gravely ill, Beatrix took over this role for this short period of time. It is evident, though, that Alistair and Beatrix have taken responsibility for supporting and protecting their mother in coping with their father.

Safety and security

All family members wanted to ensure their relatives were safe and secure, although this was not always possible. This was a significant problem, as they frequently had to deal with people (often professionals), who did not understand brain injury or the needs of their respective relatives. The views of the individuals with 'invisible deficits' were often taken at face value, and information from the family ignored. Jeanne highlighted Adam's friends, who did not protect him when he went on holiday with them.

Deidre was acutely aware of the potential risks to her father and could not rely on care home staff to provide for his needs. A bespoke support team provided consistency of care for her father, and she felt secure in the knowledge that he was safe. Laura, in contrast, feels her husband is safe with the care he is receiving.

Alistair and Beatrix did not feel safe or secure during their childhood, as they lived in fear of their father's unpredictable moods and what he might do, even though their mother provided consistent support to them over time.

Grief and losses

Relatives live with their own complex trauma, losses and grief. All contributors noted the losses that the brain injury brought and the emotional impact that this had upon them and others in their life. The nature of the grief caused by the injury was identified as complex and one that relatives generally felt very unsupported with, particularly if the injured party had made an ostensibly 'good' recovery in terms of physical abilities. The grief was identified as being endless. The losses were described as changes of role, a loss of previously held expectations and assumptions, and the loss of time and opportunity, as the family member had additional responsibilities and commitments. Contributors were able to describe their grief and recognise their losses, but noted that they felt alone with this. Their experience lead some to question the value of the life of the injured party.

Grief

As parents, Dan and Jeanne, highlighted their grief. Dan said he grieved for the life his son had lost, but as his son had changed so much, he could never properly grieve his loss. The injury was always there with him. He felt a conflict and was unsure whether to be thankful for what they had or mourn what they had lost. Jeanne said that grief was ever present for them all, as they were confronted daily through their struggles with what was happening and what had gone from their lives.

Laura said she channelled her grief, anger, frustrations and emotions into fighting for the best possible care and funding for John. Grieving started after the battle for funding was over, and this grieving continued. Laura commented, *'How do you move forwards and live your life, when you are constantly pulled back into the situation on a daily basis, whether you want to be or not?'* and *'I carry on with life, whilst always carrying the load or baggage that cannot be left behind.'* It is *'hard to remain positive and drive yourself forward'*.

Deidre lost her mother in the accident in which her father sustained his brain injury, and grieved for both her parents. She had once thought the worst thing that could have happened would have been if both her parents had died, but now fact considered it would been worse if they had both sustained a brain injury.

Ambiguous loss

Ambiguous loss is when the survivor or family members are experiencing the psychological loss of a person through some event or illness (Boss, 2006). In the case of brain injury, there is no physical death but loss of the person that the family and friends once knew. This type of loss can traumatise the survivor, friend or family member to the point where they lose all coping skills and their 'resilience' is 'lost in a frozen iceberg of grief' (Boss, 2006, p. 26). There is no closure. This continuing reminder of loss causes confusion, immobilisation and exhaustion, leading to a family member being unable to make decisions, and to make the necessary reorganisation of family roles and rules required to cope. If there is significant change in one family member, then it will impact and change the rest of the family, and this will have an effect on outcome (Maitz and Sachs, 1995).

Jeanne said, *'The son we have today is not the son I gave birth to and nurtured into a man'*. She described how the hardest loss was when she was with him, but it was not really him.

Laura talked about this ambiguous loss. She said, '*Sometimes he feels like a stranger and yet physically he is there. He looks at me as if nothing has changed*'. Laura described how her son Ben visited his father to proudly tell him of his GCSE results. Owing to the severity of John's difficulties he was unable to respond positively and congratulate his son but seemingly ignored Ben and demanded a drink. Laura said that Ben was very upset. What he wanted simply could not happen, as his father simply could not care. This was not a choice he was making. John would be unable to provide his children with the loving affirmation he would have done had the stroke not occurred.

Eliza described how her sister was not the same and how she felt she had lost her sister in the accident.

Deidre felt '*robbed*' by having her parents taken away from her and commented that while she appreciated her father was still there, he was different.

Feelings of loss

Laura has the constant feeling of being alone, as she cannot listen or share information with John or enjoy a closeness or a hug with him at the end of the day. Watching other couples, who have a closeness, or other families having fun, are constant reminders of what she has lost.

Losses are highlighted at family anniversaries or events that John cannot attend and are particularly difficult to cope with emotionally. Her son said, '*it's just like something is permanently missing from home Mum*'.

Financial losses

Grace talked about the need to financially support her family after the accident, as her mother had to give up her work to care for him.

Lost opportunities

Dan said he never knows what his son could have been and was therefore struggling with a loss of a possible future.

Laura described how she and her husband had enjoyed being parents, but they were also looking forward to spending time alone together. She lost that opportunity.

Deidre described her lost opportunities to have a family, socialise with friends and experience life in the same way as she would have done if the accident had not occurred.

Alistair talked about a *'loss of normality'*. He had difficulties knowing what a *'normal'* life was as he had missed out on so much as a child. Alistair was trying to feel comfortable undertaking activities and going on holiday with his children.

Guilt

All family members expressed guilt for different reasons. Dan felt guilty because he was not there to stop Paul from getting hurt that day. Laura reported the hardest thing was to stop feeling guilty, as she could not care for John at home, but that decision had become easier over time.

Eliza told of her feelings of guilt at not spending enough time with her sister, but also explained that she felt drained after spending any length of time with her, as she found her sister's behaviour difficult to manage.

Deidre felt guilty for sometimes wishing her father had died and when coming to the realisation that she considered it worse to have to cope with his brain injury than with his death.

Emotional challenges

Dan felt 'emotionally raw' and angry because of being unable to, as a dad, make Paul feel better or take his pain away. Dan said he felt angry with those people and organisations he could not trust, who did not have Paul's welfare as their priority. He tried shouting, but it did not work, so he learnt to manage his emotions and adapt his communication style to cope more effectively. He commented that he was *'full of sadness about how it all is'*.

Jeanne is a psychotherapist and received counselling, but she received little rehabilitation and support in caring for Adam. Adam's unpredictable and impulsive behaviours have created constant challenges. Her other children have also had emotional traumas in trying to deal with the changes in their sibling's behaviour, and their needs were unintentionally neglected, as Jeanne could not do more in the circumstances. They had no external support.

Laura said that she had fluctuating emotions, good and bad days, days of positivity and days of despair, and it was often difficult for her to know what she needed or would like. Living in the moment was still too painful. She described being on auto-pilot – she cannot remember yesterday, is often not living today, but is constantly thinking about what's happening tomorrow.

Grace has suffered from significant stress and a loss of energy since her brother's accident and these challenges have been particularly evident when demands in her life increase, and issues have arisen which have impacted on her mother's health and wellbeing.

Deidre described her emotional rollercoaster and it is noted, when working with her, that she only sought assistance from her case manager at times when she recognised her emotional responses were being challenged by difficult situations that arose relating to the care of her father.

Alistair and Beatrix were open in describing the emotional challenges they experienced throughout their childhood and how they coped.

Stress and demands

All family members described the stresses, tensions and demands they were all having to deal with, especially in the early stages after the accident. Dan acknowledged the pressure he was under and, whilst he thought he was doing very well, others around him noted his difficulties. Jeanne's story highlights how her husband and children initially tried to reduce the pressure she was under when caring for Adam, but this impacted on their own health and well-being. She, and her husband, have constantly been drawn back to try and deal with Adam's moods and unpredictable behaviour, as well as the criminal justice system, in addition to supporting Adam's children. Laura described the stresses involved in juggling her different roles in the home whilst also trying to support the needs of her husband and children.

Deidre described her emotional rollercoaster of a journey, in becoming overwhelmed, ill and emotionally unable to do anything for about five years because of having too much to do. The stresses included working, caring for her father, and worrying about all the responsibilities and organisation involved in managing her father's needs.

Grace stated they had to totally focus on the present and what needed to be done, however stressful it was.

Eliza said she felt she needed to be there to support and be available to act on her adopted sister's behalf, but this was not without its stresses, as her sister lacked insight and was challenging in her behaviour.

Burden of care

Family members often provide care and support, whether this is direct supervision, companionship, prompts/reminders or physical assistance, or interventions to reduce risks and maintain their relatives' safety. Indirect support may also be required in all aspects of their lives, organising the life of the injured person such as activities or events, accompanying their relative to appointments, dealing with practical issues, being available for guidance and problem solving, providing reassurance when emotionally challenged and giving immediate responses to crises that arise.

In addition, their injured relative is often unable to fulfil roles that they would have undertaken prior to the accident, for instance, working to support the family, providing care of children, fulfilling community roles, helping with financial and household management, providing transport, or organising leisure activities and holidays. Other members of the family have to take over these roles, in addition to providing care and support.

This burden of care can be there directly after the immediate trauma, during rehabilitation or when establishing independence in the community. If the injured relative has sustained a severe brain injury, input may be required throughout life, and this is often extremely challenging.

In their narratives, the contributors spoke of their burdens. Jeanne had worked as a psychotherapist before Adam's accident, but had to give up this role to be mother, nurse, teacher and carer, on duty day and night.

Laura commented that she experienced constant frustrations when things went wrong in the house, as John would have been able to sort them out before his stroke. She had additional work to do or would incur additional costs by calling someone in.

Eliza talked about the burden of caring that her mother carried, and explained how she never fully appreciated why her mother acted as she did on occasions, until she herself took over these responsibilities after her death.

Grace described how her brother had obsessive compulsive disorder as a consequence of his brain injury. He did not like people entering the house. His mother or sister had to manage everything carefully, with patience, time and preparation to manage any fears he had before work could be undertaken in the home.

Embarrassment and rejection

Younger children and siblings were more likely to be embarrassed by the odd parent/sibling behaviours, than parents or spouses, who were older and potentially more able to handle challenging situations. The children and siblings described feelings of embarrassment and rejection from their parents, siblings, schoolfriends and members of the public.

Alistair and Beatrix described how their father's behaviour was embarrassing to them when they were children, and how difficult it was to introduce him to anybody or explain to their friends why he was like he was. Their father's behaviour changed other people's attitudes towards them, and they were rejected from normal social activities and events as a consequence of this.

Eliza described feelings of rejection and resentment, as all of her parents' attention was focused on her sister. Fortunately, she was of an age when she could talk to her mother about this issue and her feelings dissipated. Eliza and her mother remained very close and were always there for each other.

Trust

In Dan's narrative he describes how he learnt to trust people even though he did not always believe or agree with them, and talked about the professional team becoming part of his family, which was a form of acceptance for him.

Jeanne did not have support from professionals for the rehabilitation and care of her son for a very long time. She did not have the opportunity to develop relationships and trust anyone to care for her son as there was nobody available for her.

Laura developed trusting relationships with the rehabilitation and care staff who worked with her husband, but lost faith in health care professionals, especially those from the CCG, as promises were made to her but not fulfilled.

Deidre could not trust professionals or carers who lacked understanding of brain injury, as they could not see what was required and how the care had to be provided to ensure her father's safety and comfort. She was reassured that her father had good care from the bespoke support work team who knew him well. She trusted and respected them.

Resilience

All of the contributors demonstrated their resilience, under pressure, to support and provide care for their injured relatives over a very long period of time. They continue to do so. This resilience has been achieved because they have a perceived duty to help their loved one and want them to be safe and supported. They are often challenged because they are continually under extreme pressure and are often without choices or alternatives, morally and practically, to do anything other than what they are already doing to their best ability, i.e. acting in their relative's best interests.

Dan was particularly challenged when other family members and professionals did not appreciate his son's 'invisible deficits'. He had to go to court to protect his son's interests and protect him from himself (as he lacked insight), and highlight the potential risks to his children. His social worker thought he could be left alone to care for two children under the age of 5, when he was unable to initiate any 'novel actions' or safely respond in everyday situations.

Laura described the need to do things properly on behalf of her husband. She found it was easier to be strong and fight when you are doing it for somebody else rather than yourself. She could not believe how she got through the fight, when she had been mourning the loss of her husband but commented, *'something inside gets you through'*.

Grace described how her resilience fluctuated and, although over time, her feelings had changed to resignation and acceptance, she still found the challenges difficult to cope with.

Communication

Communication appears to be key, as is evident in many of the contributors' narratives. When positive, it creates trust, understanding and collaboration, but when it breaks down, issues often arise.

Dan described communication issues with the professionals, as he did not appreciate the language used or their approaches. He considered they were making assumptions about knowing his son, when he was the 'expert'. He and the professionals managed to create a therapeutic relationship and the collaboration to ensure communication was effective. Dan described how he learned to communicate in a way that others could clearly hear what he had to say.

Jeanne had no support and was so overwhelmed and immersed in Adam's care that communication with her other children became less effective and they suffered health issues as a consequence.

Laura made a point of creating opportunities to communicate with her children about all the issues, and she developed good communication with the therapists and care staff who were working with her husband. She had key communication difficulties with the CCG representatives, who increased her feelings of guilt at not having her husband home and, for whatever reason, could not hear what her husband's needs were.

The siblings, Eliza and Grace, have had limited communication with professionals. Eliza's mother took primary responsibility for communicating about her daughter and Eliza only took over when she died. Grace's brother has no friends and very limited professional input.

Deidre was an effective communicator for her father. Beatrix said that their mother did not want them to talk to others, i.e. friends or teachers, about their father's behaviour or what was going on in the family home. This meant that Beatrix and Alistair were restricted in whom they could talk to about the situation when they were young. They are now able to communicate openly and honestly.

Feeling marginalised and discrepancies of fit

Dan and Laura both described feeling marginalised by rehabilitation and health care professionals; particularly in multidisciplinary team meetings when professionals described what their relatives' problems were and what they were doing, without appreciating who their 'loved one' was, and without explanation or reference to the family member for their views. Rehabilitation professionals took over the decision-making on their relatives' behalf, despite the fact that they were the person responsible for supporting their family member. In this situation relatives were able to provide feedback (in some form or other), so the professionals could establish positive therapeutic relationships. They both learnt medical terminology and professionals' language and gained an understanding of the systems and processes required for rehabilitation and care of their injured relative. As a nurse, Deidre already had this knowledge and fully appreciated how difficult it was for family members who did not know who to go to or how the system worked.

Laura noted support groups she had attended in her narrative but described how the family did not feel they fitted into any of these groups. Deidre also described the problem of 'not fitting in' or being a 'square peg in a round hole' as, due to her unique position of both a professional and family member, she did not have shared experiences with other family members.

Attitudes and understanding of others

Family members said their friends had dwindled away, as they themselves were overwhelmed with different stresses and demands on their time, working, caring for and supporting their injured relative, and keeping their families together, let alone managing all the normal household jobs. Limited time and opportunities for maintaining their social life was evident in all circumstances.

All family members described how many people they met had no understanding of brain injury or what their lives were really like. They had to learn to cope with this fact.

Dan and Jeanne both commented that people frequently said how lucky their sons were, because they looked normal. Such people had no appreciation of how untrue Dan and Jeanne thought that view was, and how this merely served to highlighted outsiders' lack of understanding and was no consolation at all.

Laura said that when people asked her how she was, they were not really interested. If she did explain, they did not know what to say or how to respond. She described how these people acted in a way that they thought was best for her rather than ask her what she needed. However, she did acknowledge it was often difficult for her to know what she needed or would like. Laura also commented on being watched as a family when they all went out together.

Deidre described how difficult it was for her friends to understand the difficulties she had in caring for her father until later, when they started to care for their own elderly relatives.

Alistair and Beatrix described how other members of their family and friends did not understand their father's injuries and thought he had a mental illness.

Changes in roles and relationships

Each family member has their own unique thread of recognition with their family member and within each particular relationship in the family. These unique relationships change after a family member sustains a brain injury and this also affects the family dynamics. From that time on, the family unit has to change and adjust in accordance with the altered needs of the injured relative, with altered roles, relationships and interdependencies. Each of our contributors experienced the injury to their loved one in a unique context, a context which has affected and shaped their experiences and is central to it.

Relationships with their relative

Dan has always had a close relationship with Paul but since Paul's injury it has taken 17 years to re-establish it. Dan constantly has to monitor how Paul is doing and ascertain if he needs to intervene for any reason to ensure all are working with him, to enable him to do what he desires and needs to do. Dan described how they had managed to, Paul, his wife and two children, despite the brain injury.

Jeanne and her husband re-mortgaged their home to purchase another nearby for Adam. This did not relieve their pressures, as Jeanne had to support him at his home when he was drinking to excess, became depressed and suicidal. Adam was given a suspended sentence after being aggressive to an ex-girlfriend. Jeanne and her husband continue to provide ongoing support for Adam, as he lacks insight into his capabilities and has poor executive skills. He has limited external support, so they still have to step in to deal with all crises.

John was Laura's main support before the accident and at the time when she needed him most, emotionally and practically, he was no longer there. She felt alone. She continues to visit, take him out and support him as much as she is able.

Grace copes with her brother's unpredictable changes in moods and contamination OCD, and, despite receiving no appreciation from her brother, maintains the support to her mother and brother, and ensures her brother's needs are met.

Eliza listens to her sister's frustrations and provides advocacy and support for her. Frances is resident in a specialist long-stay rehabilitation facility, due to the severity of her behavioural difficulties. Eliza takes her sister on days out or to concerts occasionally, but limits her input, as she feels impatient when hearing the same comments repeatedly. She always has to be careful in what she says, in case it provokes her sister to have a temper tantrum.

Deidre became a parent to her father overnight, on the same day that she lost her mother. She had learnt to manage her father's difficult behaviours following his ABI, for instance, wandering off, repeated questions, impulsive behaviours and inappropriate comments, but at the time of her contribution to the book, her father was physically deteriorating, fully dependent on others for all of his needs, and end of life care was being discussed.

Alistair and Beatrix have had a lifetime of coping with their father, of having to be responsive to their father's demands and dealing with his behaviour, and totally missed out on the normal father/child relationship.

Alistair described how he had to be a grown-up from an early age and protect his mother and sister. Beatrix reported the role changed as they grew older. Christine was their protector in the early years and then it changed; as she and Alistair got older, they protected their mother.

Relationships and dynamics within the immediate family over time

It is evident how, in most cases, the bonds within the family relationships became stronger, as a consequence of the shared experiences. Coping with the trauma, dealing with the consequences and providing ongoing love and support through crises appears to have forged a 'closeness in working together' in dealing with their injured relative and coping with the world.

PARENTS

Dan said, '*I am his dad and I'm obligated to be his dad until the day I die*', and it was his duty to care for and protect his son. He believed parenting was a full-time role (support, prompts, guiding and reassurance) and a parent's commitment to their children should be lifelong, for as long as they were needed. The parent–child relationship is strong, and inherent in this is acknowledged acceptance of values and roles they would normally undertake.

Dan talked about Paul's accident and how it had changed the whole family, and how it had taken 17 years to get back to the point where they have a father–son relationship. Paul agrees with everything anyone says to him. There were conflicts because of the differing perceptions between family members of Paul's needs. There were times when Dan's acrimonious relationship with his ex-wife was exacerbated. For instance, Dan described how his views of what his son needed were in conflict with the views of his ex-wife, Paul's mother, and battle lines were drawn. The court sided with Dan's opinion, but this was undoubtedly a time of great stress when the stakes were very high. Fortunately, and perhaps surprisingly, Dan has managed to achieve a good working relationship with his ex-wife, as he recognised that this was in Paul's best interests.

Dan talked about the support and strength of close others, especially Anna, his wife, who had helped him to carry on at times when he felt particularly overwhelmed and emotionally challenged. Anna reflected on issues, took useful action on his son's behalf and maintained the family unit, when Dan could not emotionally do this. He described how his family became closer and tighter than ever before because of the brain injury.

Dan and Jeanne have not only had their adult children suddenly become dependent on them again, but then, after re-establishing a degree of independence, develop new (and unstable) relationships with vulnerable partners and become parents themselves. Dan and Jeanne have more dependents to feel responsible for, with additional anxieties and burdens in their lives, because of their relatives' limited abilities. However, this is also a new and very positive focus for their attention, as they are in the different role of grandparents.

Jeanne received counselling for the traumas she had to cope with, for instance, being at the scene of the accident, dealing with the consequences of this, and grieving for a friend who died shortly after Adam's accident. The whole household revolved around Adam, as he had unpredictable behaviour, used inappropriate language and displayed significant verbal and physical aggression. Jeanne initially was too overwhelmed to cope and look after everyone in the family and she had to put her other children's needs on the back burner. She could not leave Adam and his younger brother alone together, as Adam would hit him. Her other children have had difficulties since that time. Adam's brother started to overeat and was bullied at school, and he withdrew. Adam's sister was at the scene of the accident and saw her brother fighting for his life, and she gave up eating, as Adam had gone off to get food when the accident occurred. She now lives abroad and has ongoing health issues.

SPOUSE

Whilst all marriages/partnerships are unique, the spouse is an intimate soulmate who shares experiences and provides companionship. Collaboration over time establishes the role for each partner, and routines and systems in the family home are formed for their unique family unit.

After a brain injury, the spouse can have competing issues to manage, for instance with their relative's condition, their rehabilitation and needs, and their children's responses to the changed circumstances, in addition to taking over the roles that their injured partner would have otherwise undertaken.

Laura lost the partner she had relied on and had to bring up their children alone, which is not what she would have wished for. She had to be there to support her family and their emotions through their experiences. Her children now have a deep appreciation for people with mental and physical disabilities.

The conflicting issues for Christine were whether to remain with her husband and care for him, or leave him. Christine has a strong religious faith and felt she needed to fulfil her marriage vows *'for better or worse'*. She knew that her husband could not manage alone, or independently and, without the family support, he would neglect himself and possibly die. She also thought that if she left him they would have financial insecurities that would impact on the children's health and well-being.

SIBLINGS

Siblings are often the forgotten members of the family when it comes to survival of family members after brain injury. Parents or spouses usually take responsibility for the care of their injured relatives. Depending on the age of siblings at the time, they may be taken away from the family home and supported by other relatives or friends immediately after the accident, or they might not be living at home or be present during the crisis. The siblings might not only have the challenges of coping with their brother or sister after the accident, but their needs may be overlooked because their parents are preoccupied with their injured sibling and the ongoing stresses that arise.

What is unique and important about siblings is that they are possibly the only family members who will be alive for most of their injured relative's lifetime, from childhood to old age. They are the group that, if their relative does not have a partner or children, may be expected to be their next of kin and responsible for them, if their parents are no longer around to support their injured relative.

The impact on Adam's siblings was significant. They suffered health and psychological problems after his accident, which affected their development and continue to affect their wellbeing.

Eliza's mother provided most of her sister's care for many years, but her father never understood his daughter's brain injury and behavioural changes. He could never talk about his daughter. Eliza's mother said she would have divorced her husband if the case manager had not been available to support her. Eliza described taking over the responsibility of supporting her sister after her parents died. Her injured sister is currently in a long-stay rehabilitation setting, after a community placement failed, and she now has less direct responsibility for ensuring her health and wellbeing.

Grace's bond with her mother is very close and they talked about their 'partnership' in dealing with issues that arose.

CHILDREN

It will depend on the child's age and experiences, previous relationships with their parents and the nature of their injured parent's condition, as to the degree of responsibility and involvement they have in supporting their injured relative and other parent.

Deidre described how one of her roles was of keeping the family together by supporting her siblings and their families and informing them as to her father's condition.

Parents, like Laura, included their children in the process, sensitively informing them of the heartbreaking news of their father's condition and of any changes that were likely to help them better understand and manage the situation.

Jeanne had more difficulty in supporting her children. They withdrew, as they did not want to increase their mother's burden, but this meant their own needs were neglected.

Injured parents who have particular behaviours, for instance mood disturbances, inconsistent responses, unexplainable losses of temper and control, and lack of empathy, create difficulties for their offspring. Forgetting important information, doing strange things, or making the child feel stupid when unable to do simple activities are just some of the issues that can arise. This creates a home environment which can lead to behaviours such as withdrawal, fear, anxiety, acting out and aggression.

Beatrix described how she had to follow her father's instructions immediately, as she was scared of what might happen if she responded negatively. Alistair also reported being blamed for things he had not done. Both were fearful of their father having behavioural outbursts, losing his temper and hitting them.

Alistair had some understanding of the differences in his father after the accident, whereas Beatrix did not. Recognition of how their father was different emerged over time. When their father unpredictably responded to them or rejected them, this created conflicts and emotional challenges for them to cope with.

Alistair and Beatrix highlighted their need for safety and security, which was not possible until they grew older and could stand up to their father together. As they have developed over the years, they have supported, challenged, protected and guided their father, and worked around the issues, as far as they have been able.

Alistair and Beatrix have a very close relationship and they learnt very quickly to protect each other, and continue to do so. Beatrix said they would always look out for each other and go above and beyond to help one another. Beatrix lives in the family home with her parents, and Alistair lives with his wife and two children. Christine is supportive of both children and is now the main support for her husband, although she tries to keep out of his way as much as she can.

Differences in views between family members continue to be apparent for the younger children, although there is no acrimony or regret.

Alistair said that he was positive they had managed to remain together as a family against all odds.

OTHER FAMILY MEMBERS, GRANDPARENTS, GRANDCHILDREN, ETC.

Jeanne said her extended family did not visit or understand what the family were coping with. Once she had developed a better understanding of her son's condition, she had been able to educate others, in particular their granddaughters, and enable them to understand why the dad they love so much is so embarrassing.

Beatrix described how their relationship with their grandparents became 'strained' and the grandparents did little to help them. She and Alistair adored their grandparents, but they found out later that their father could not cope with their grandad teaching them skills he could not teach them himself.

Reflections and living with the future

Dan described how for him, '*it never ends, there's no getting away from it, no relief and it will never get better. It hurt then, and it hurts now but I have to accept where things are now – nothing I can do about it – have to crack on with it*'. He acknowledges how his son's brain injury had positively changed him as a person, as he had learnt skills like patience, tolerance, humility, eloquence in his communication, and to cope more effectively with situations. This has changed his life. Dan said, '*in all the bad bits, there are always little wins, dark times but there will be little bits of light*'.

Dan wants to be the best dad he can and perceives that, if he is the best dad, then by default Paul will be the best dad he can be. Dan knows that people (including professionals) do not see Paul's 'invisible problems' and that he will have to provide evidence regarding his son's condition to anyone new that comes into their lives.

Jeanne said, '*Life does not take you on the journey you would want.*' Adam lacks insight, has executive deficits and is impulsive: he has fluctuations of mood and drinks to excess and has been involved in the criminal justice system. Jeanne has had to support Adam within all aspects of society previously unknown to her. She is aware that issues are highly likely to arise in the future, and that she will have to be intervene as and when required.

Laura has needed to challenge funding agencies and has built her life around her visits to her husband. She has core values that keep her going and is learning to appreciate what she has. She has difficulty in adjusting to a different life and is just taking one day, or even one hour at a time to be able to move forward. She also described her life as 'living in limbo', 'frozen in time' and 'life moves on, but I am not moving with it'.

Grace dreads the time in the not-too-distant future when her mother is not going to be there anymore and is aware that she may well be required to do more when her mother dies.

Alistair and Beatrix highlighted that the issues with their father do not go away and they will always have to carefully manage and supervise their father, when he sees his grandchildren.

Coping with the rehabilitation services/professionals – help or hinder

All of the families shared their experiences of professionals lacking an understanding of the consequences of the brain injury and the needs of the relatives.

Early stages

One issue in the early stages is that professionals cannot give the families the information required to reassure them that all will be alright. The professionals can be supportive in helping them understand what they are doing to help their relative, giving them time to talk about and deal with practical issues, and providing them with as much comfort, as possible, for instance, places to sit or stay, places to get food and drink, and access to information, as and when it becomes available.

Jeanne mentioned the doctors saying Adam would need a miracle to survive and the question was raised as to whether the machines would need to be turned off or not. Adam survived. Jeanne was told, when Adam was in a vegetative state, not to expect much more due to the enormity of his injuries.

Laura remembered the manner of the professionals when they were talking about her partner. She appreciated the consultant, who was 'open, honest and caring' and how he had asked her if there was anything else he could do to help.

However, in contrast to this, Eliza recalled how a nurse made a cruel comment, 'Pray she dies', to her parents when her sister was in the Intensive Care Unit.

Rehabilitation

When the rehabilitation professionals told Dan he ought to be doing things differently with Paul, he responded negatively, as he knew his son better than the professionals. He did not want to say anything negative in front of Paul, as Dan did not want him to feel bad for the benefit of these professionals. Dan found the professionals overly intrusive and, although he wanted to trust them, he was very nervous about being able to do so. As a parent, being able to trust someone to do their job and let them look after his child was extremely difficult and it was challenging for him to accept input.

Laura had a supportive multidisciplinary team working with her husband and she could raise any issues she needed to with her husband's keyworker. The MDT also reinforced how they had learnt from Laura and John. Laura did not trust the assessor from the Continuing Healthcare, who did not even give her the respect of remembering her name, made her feel guilty for not having her husband at home, and downgraded the scoring so John did not get funding. This was even though the multidisciplinary team agreed he should qualify. Laura had to complain that the assessment had not followed due process, contacted her MP and had to wait two months for any response from the CCG. Then she had to arrange a meeting with the Director of Quality for the CCG. Fortunately, this person listened to her.

Grace described how the professionals (the rare ones they have had contact with) wanted to try and fix the situation, whereas Grace and her mother wanted a framework of rehabilitation relevant to Henry's needs.

Deidre highlighted incidents where she did not to trust the professionals involved in her father's care, as they lacked understanding of brain injury and did not know how to manage him – even those who were supposed to know what to do. She highlighted a psychiatrist, who gave large doses of drugs which caused her father to get worse, and a nurse who blamed her for her father's behaviour in the rehabilitation setting when he wandered off or collected other resident's belongings. She was also frustrated by the lack of communication from the professionals; for instance, a failure to provide rehabilitation and care plans.

Longer-term relationships with professionals

Dan had to fight professionals for Paul's disability to be recognised and to get the support he needed. Professionals (and others) did not see or understand what his son's problems were. He had to deal with conflicting opinions of professionals, as they could not agree in respect of Paul's support needs, and he found this confusing and frustrating. Professionals spoke a different language, which he had to learn, and then he had to deal with statutory systems, like Health and Social Services, solicitors, Court of Protection, medical specialists, therapists and social workers, which he had no experience of before – they were challenging for him to deal with.

Jeanne has been let down from the outset. She was not provided with information about brain injury, rehabilitation approaches or support to know what to do when Adam was discharged home. She did not receive any support from the social worker who visited her and who on one occasion did not even wait to see Adam. On another visit, Adam was accused of being lazy and was informed that they could offer nothing unless his parents made him homeless. The social workers were not trained in brain injury.

Jeanne did not receive any support for 10 years and then only received help from the mental health team when Adam was depressed and suicidal. Adam was allocated a CPN and funded for six weeks' rehabilitation at Headway. After Adam got into trouble again and required reconstruction surgery after a fight, he became more depressed and afraid to go out. Jeanne sought a referral to a neuropsychologist and then waited nine months for an appointment.

Laura has found it challenging watching others take care of John, and being told his likes and dislikes, when she knows him best. She has had to learn to accept and step back from these everyday situations.

Eliza described how easily professionals were fooled at interview by the way her sister presented rather than ask others about what she did and how she characteristically behaved.

Grace commented on how professionals would listen to her brother but not to other members of the family, when they were the ones suffering significant stress from coping with his challenging behaviour.

Dan, Alistair and Beatrix commented on the positive support they received from their independent case manager, a role funded by litigation and rarely available via statutory services.

Professionals working with professionals

Deidre defined the positive and negative aspects of her professional and personal role in coping with her father's rehabilitation and care. She had knowledge, skills and experience but little support to help her cope with her emotions. Whenever Deidre was in a support group, she switched into a professional mode to support others. She learnt to split off from her professional role as a nurse when dealing with medical or nursing issues as a family member.

Jeanne's professional status as a psychotherapist meant she was not viewed as requiring any support or help. It took ten years, from after acute rehabilitation, before they received any outside help.

Dan noted that his experience of dealing with professionals changed his approach to his own career, helped develop his style of communication, and that he had progressed to a senior management level partly as a consequence of these positive changes.

References

Boss, P. 2006. *Loss, trauma and resilience: therapeutic work with ambiguous loss*. New York: W.W. Norton.

Maitz, E.A., & Sachs, P.R. 1995. Treating families of individuals with traumatic brain injury from a family systems perspective. *Journal of Head Trauma Rehabilitation*, 10.

Chapter 9

What may help?

Our contributors all agreed to write their story for this book so that their experiences could be shared, and their hard-fought wisdom and practical ways of finding resilience could benefit others. In this chapter their recommendations are reviewed in the context of the current literature and the authors' knowledge and experience. Recommendations are made as to what might help support families of individuals with severe brain injury.

It is fully recognised that everyone is unique, with different lifestyles and distinct ways of coping; there will be no one solution that fits all. Specialist resources are patchy around the UK, as is the professionals' understanding and support for families after brain injury. The provision of appropriate support to families is very dependent on the appreciation of the trauma that family members suffer over time. If a serious brain injury happened to any of us or a member of our family, could we predict what kind of support would be available to us, and whether people would be there to help in the long term?

The recommendations are included in these general points, as identified by the contributors:

Safety, security and feeling supported

The contributors all expressed the value of feeling safe and supported, and having a degree of control of their life. This helped them cope with the chaos and uncertainties that were present. Without this security, everything became overwhelming and unsustainable.

Feeling 'safe' for the contributors meant having relevant, factual information about their relative, especially in the early stages of recovery, so they knew at all times what was going on. The contributors wanted to be heard and valued. They expressed the need to be recognised and acknowledged as the experts, as they knew their relative better than anyone else. They wanted to feel involved and validated as being integral to the rehabilitation/support process.

The contributors expressed how having everyday structures and stability helped them maintain normal life routines and the status quo, as far as possible, not only for themselves but also for other members of the family. The contributors acknowledged that having money aided security, for instance, in the provision of care and support.

Feeling 'supported' meant having practical and emotional support, as and when required (rather than at a time of convenience to others), to reduce the pressures of excessive demands and undue stresses, when constantly having to adapt to different situations. The parents and spouse acknowledged the juggling just to cope with the basics, like shopping, housework, childcare, whilst managing their own emotions, in order to keep everything going. Family carers valued the support they received from other family members, friends, and the kindness of others, but also from people who had shared experiences.

Timely, relevant, and valid information

Generic information on brain injury is available on the Internet, in publications, articles and books and from handouts and pamphlets from charitable organisations like Headway, local Headway groups, Children's Brain Injury Trust (CBIT) Children's Trust, Brains Matter, British Association of Brain Injury Case Managers (BABICM), the Brain Injury Social Work Group, Encephalitis Society, the Meningitis charity, Different Strokes and the Stroke Association. There are also telephone chat lines and opportunities for web chats and webinars to learn more information.

Although generic information is valuable, additional information and support is required to help families understand more precisely what is happening to their relative and the reasons for the changes they observe. Families of individuals with severe brain injury highlighted the need to know information, as this contributed greatly in reducing intense feelings of anxiety and distress (Bond et al., 2003).

Immediately after the accident, families are rarely ever prepared or fully informed about everything. Those professionals involved are focused on dealing with life and death decisions, and attentive to maintaining the life of their relative. Molter identified that, at this time, families wanted to be given hope, and to know people around them cared about their relative. They needed to be near their relative and to know, when not present at the hospital, that they would be called at home immediately if there were any changes in their relative's condition. The families wanted to know their relatives' prognosis, to have their questions answered honestly and to be given specific facts concerning their relative's progress. Families wished to see their relative frequently, have feedback about their relative's condition at least once a day, and to be given information with explanations that were understandable. (Molter, 1979, Fins and Solomon, 2001).

Specificity of information becomes more important over time, as families experience particular issues with their relative in everyday life. They need individual attention and support to make sense of their experience. Specific information about one's relative needs to be created over time in the context of a more general understanding of the effects of brain injury. This awareness arises through conversations with knowledgeable others (be they professionals or peers) and by integrating information to create a person-centred and bespoke understanding of the situation. Families need to create a cohesive and bespoke narrative over time about what has happened to their relative with a brain injury, and to understand the reasons for the changes they observe in their relative in respect to behaviour, cognitions, emotions and lifestyle. Families need help to do this.

Reducing burden of care

Sometimes it is the 'little things' that can make a massive difference to families in reducing the burden of care. Family and friends being on their side, being there and available for support or to take over, as and when required, can help. Practical assistance can take pressure off, for instance, care/support, transportation, taking care of children or other dependents and preparing meals; and financial support can also aid the situation. The contributors acknowledged the need to develop and maintain a balanced lifestyle, with social opportunities, in order to maintain their emotional well-being in the long term.

Many families have no choice but to support their injured relative when discharged from hospital without warning or preparation for the care required over time. Whereas some families are happy with this arrangement, others do not feel comfortable undertaking care, as this changes the relationship with their relative, whether this is the spouse, parent, siblings or children. The latter families may want their injured relative to have the opportunity for increased independence and background support provided from trusted support workers, whom they oversee to ensure the injured individual is safe and has a reasonable quality of life.

No-one welcomes a trauma that changes the entire trajectory of a person's life. It is important for the longevity of the family unit that those who are overwhelmed by their burden of care are facilitated to feel more in control of and engaged in their lives. Family members who feel hopeless, helpless and passive need the appropriate support to become proactive and self-determined and involved in the rehabilitation process (Ponsford et al., 2003). Saying and achieving this are two different things.

Family members often require more assistance or support over time, as the care of individuals with brain injury can be overwhelming, exhausting, debilitating and challenging. Families need time and respite from providing care, especially as the burden of care increases (Brooks and McKinlay, 1983), and families whose injured relative has behaviour problems are considered to have special needs and require specific skills to deal with them (Junque, 1997). Injured relatives with behaviour issues, associated with executive deficits, lack of insight, impulsivity, increased anxiety and aggression, are extremely difficult to manage within family units, in comparison with those who have severe physical deficits. If structure and support cannot be provided or maintained for those with behaviour problems, the individuals can develop further problems associated with a chaotic lifestyle, often including alcohol and drug abuse and criminal activities.

Creating support for the injured relative can be a stressful process, as establishing funding and finding the 'right' person or people, whom relatives trust and feel comfortable with in their home, takes time. Support workers (carers or buddies) can be available via agencies or direct recruitment, and there are pros and cons in making the decision for each option. Guidance for recruiting, employing, training, managing and paying support workers is often required, as this can be complex to ensure the requirements of employment law are fulfilled. Some experienced case managers have the resources to undertake this process.

Stress and mental health issues

Laura highlighted the importance of maintaining a sense of self: '*Be kind to yourself*' and '*have strong core values, as it helps to get you through*'.

None of us are any use to anyone else if we are burnt out. It is not surprising family members experience high levels of stress in the context of being responsive towards the needs of the injured relative, and the differing coping styles of each family member, as well as the many other demands. Relatives describe their experience during periods of high stress as *'living from one minute to the next'*, *'desperately holding on'* and *'seeking normality'*, whilst being buffeted by the ups and downs of life. Family members become used to responding to immediate demands to manage the injured relative, whilst placing their own, and also sometimes other family members' needs, on the backburner. They are just surviving and do not have the time, attention or opportunity to deal with more.

Some family members may be observers or involved in and have injuries from the same accident as their relative. Relatives can develop post- traumatic stress disorder, anxiety and depression. They may experience a range of symptoms such as increased arousal and alertness, poor sleep pattern, exhaustion, depleted energy reserves, poor nutritional intake, emotional lability including increased sensitivity, tearfulness, intolerance, irritability and aggression, loss of self-identity and negative thoughts, rumination and disassociation. A cycle of despair may develop in which the person may get stuck and unable to move forward in the absence of appropriate therapeutic input and support.

Tyerman provides some wise precautionary words. *'It is vital not to treat relatives as patients requiring treatment'* (Tyerman, 2008, p. 25). An overly clinical approach may be interpreted negatively, and families may need a light touch and a flexible, open-door approach.

Supporting family members in recognising the importance of being aware of their own needs and looking after themselves is essential to help them maintain the resilience required to support their relative over time. When family members are overly stressed and under extreme pressure, their level of physiological arousal increases, and they become less efficient. A variety of sensory and physical therapies have been shown to be effective in reducing stress and enhancing well-being, for example massage, yoga, t'ai chi, swimming and other sports. It is extremely important for family members to have time for themselves in order to feel as if they have a degree of control over events. They may need supporting to establish a regular leisure pursuit and make it happen. Mindfulness can help some: for others it makes them more anxious; having a hobby, social group, massage or physical activity works best. No one solution fits all.

Relatives experience a wide variety of emotions at different stages in the recovery process, and the needs of the family change over time depending on the circumstances they are in. It has been suggested that families should ideally have clinicians well-versed in brain injury and family therapy (Laroi, 2003).

Family members can find support groups and various psychological therapies beneficial, but the understanding of brain injury is an important factor in the provision of any interventions. These therapies include individual and supportive counselling, psychotherapy, couples' relationship therapy (Kreutzer, 2010), Cognitive-Behavioural Therapy (CBT), Acceptance and Commitment Therapy (ACT), Eye Movement Deensitization and Reprocessing Therapy (EMDR), family therapy, family and parental training (Ducharme, 2002) and support groups (professionally-organised and peer support groups) (Tyerman, 2008, Kreutzer, 2002, 2009).

For family members who have clinically diagnosed anxiety or depression, medical management with anxiolytics or anti-depressants can help to manage the symptoms in association with other psychological therapies.

When working with family members who have a diagnosis of post-traumatic stress disorder, it is important for this to be carefully managed by specialists, so traumas and emotions are not negatively retriggered by the therapeutic interventions.

Considering the needs of all family members

All family members have unique relationships and shared experiences, with co-dependencies on each other. A brain injury does not just happen to one person but affects the whole family, and each family member may need support to manage these changes. The uncertainties of 'not knowing' and fluctuating feelings of hope and despair continues as time goes on, until the long-term deficits and ongoing changes become evident. Sometimes the emotional reserves can be found for this to be managed within a strong family unit, but there are times when it can impact the long-term well-being of individual family members and the integrity of the family unit.

Within the immediate and extended family, increased distress can develop if there is a lack of understanding about the individual with the brain injury. Misunderstandings, misinterpretations and conflict can arise, which can be destructive to family communication and relationships. These issues are more likely to happen when individual members of the family are exhausted from caring for their relative, are under high levels of stress, suffer from overwhelming grief and are generally less able to cope emotionally with the uncertainties in their life. The contributors described how beneficial it was to have clarity of family roles and what needed to be done to prevent any family member becoming overburdened, overwhelmed and resentful about having to deal with too many demands.

Conflicts over perceived family roles or responsibilities after a traumatic accident are known to occur. For instance, maintaining support to nurture, guide and support their children is often central to the parents' lives. Spouses/partners have intimate, personal and sexual relationships. On occasions, conflict can occur when there are differences in opinion, and both spouse and parents believe they should be responsible for making decisions and providing care. When parents or spouses are overwhelmed, other children or family members may feel unable to do anything to help, or feel rejected, which may seriously affect their own health and ability to cope in everyday life. Performance at school and relationships with friends are just some aspects of their life that may suffer.

In these situations, specialists with knowledge and understanding can provide information, support and guidance about the relative with the brain injury. They can acknowledge the issues and potentially reduce frictions associated with misunderstandings, in order to negotiate ways forward with all concerned in the best interests of both the relative with the brain injury and the family members. The sharing of views and opinions can be supportive in creating a positive approach to family decision-making. As mentioned above, specific therapeutic interventions can be invaluable for individual family members but also together in family therapy, if required.

Parents

The feelings of parents seemed to be typified in the views of the mother and father contributing to this book, as would be expected because of their long-term relationship. '*Your child is yours. You know your child best and are acting in their best interests*'. '*Do whatever it takes and deal with situations in your own unique way, if this helps you cope*'.

Many parents feel a deep sense of guilt and shame in being unable to fulfil their role as a parent to keep their child safe. Parents share their child's losses, not only for aspects of their personality and abilities that have changed, but also for the loss of the child's future prospects, career, potential relationships, marriage, children and the like. Parents are the only family members (apart from possibly grandparents) where the nurturing, dependent relationship is an inherent part of their role. The changes in abilities and behaviour after a brain injury increase dependency and vulnerabilities. Some parents take back this responsibility to care for their child, even when they are adults.

Over time, parents become aware that they will not be there for their child in the long term. They may have expected support from their injured child as they grew older, which is no longer a possibility, and instead may be left caring for their child without support in their old age. Some parents fear what will happen to their relative after they die. Sometimes this responsibility can be effectively passed on to other family members (siblings or children) but, due to the nature of brain injury, there are occasions when this may not be possible. Parents may not want the same burden of care transferred to their other children.

As time and their deteriorating health becomes apparent, it is important to determine the care and support requirements the parents would like for their child after their death. This may not be a subject parents will want to think about. Experience shows there is a sense of relief if the topic is openly discussed at the right time: parents need to know what can be done to support their child in their absence, and who will make decisions on their behalf and ensure the care they know their child requires is provided. This type of conversation can only occur in the context of trust, which has been gradually built up over time with someone they feel understands the issues.

Spouses/partners

Unique to the spouses' relationship is the sharing of intimacy, sexual relationships and more personal emotions. After a brain injury many spouses/partners describe how their relationship changes from that of mutual interdependency of roles and relationships within the family unit to one of carer. This occurs in the context of additional demands on their time for maintaining and supporting the family, coping with changes in finances and increased family roles. It is known that the stress, especially on less established relationships, increases the risks of the marriage/partnership ending.

Spouses/partners may benefit from exploring their feelings with someone who understands brain injury. This can support the development of practical ways of understanding and addressing issues that arise in the relationship. Specific marital therapy has been shown to be effective in supporting individuals with brain injury and their partners to express their feelings together (Kreutzer et al., 2009). Within this safe space, it may also be possible to explore aspects of the relationship, which may need to change in a way that will work for both partners. Laura stressed the importance of being able to acknowledge and express changes in her feelings, i.e. being a loving person but not in love with her partner. This helped her achieve *'peace of mind'*.

If spouses/partners separate, this may be mutually accepted and understood, or it can become acrimonious and difficult to manage (and anything in between). Spouses may have fears about leaving, because of financial insecurity, not having anywhere to live, or fears about being able to cope alone. Many spouses feel guilty, especially if they cannot cope with the situation and have concerns about how their injured partner will manage without his or her support. Alternative arrangements may be sought, as the decision to leave or stay may be dependent on who will be able or available to care for their spouse, and whether additional resources in the way of care and support are available for them. On occasions, a crisis occurs, when the spouse cannot take any more and leaves abruptly without any plans in place, or alternatively when physical or mental health issues of the caring 'spouse' become the priority.

Issues of arrangement for children and child access can be especially tricky to deal with, particularly if the person with the brain injury has executive deficits, lack of insight or anger issues. Safety of the children is paramount, and having someone available (family or professional) who has an understanding of brain injury can be invaluable in determining whether the individual has the capacity and the capability to look after the child, with or without support. Facilitating safe child care arrangements is essential and needs to work for all.

Siblings

The sibling contributors made the following recommendations: '*Protect yourself*', '*Be accepting of them as they are*' and '*Be the person on their side*'.

Having a sibling with a traumatic brain injury can result in both profound and enduring negative or positive life changes for the non-injured siblings. Siblings have been reported to have mixed emotions towards their relative with the brain injury. In a study by Degeneffe, siblings highlighted feelings of anger at not having a normal childhood, guilt for surviving, resentment about losses, mourning for their sibling, and a fear of violent behaviour. Siblings are known to be sensitive to others' perceptions of their injured sibling. For instance, they may feel embarrassed, angry and protective when their sibling exhibits disinhibited behaviour, makes inappropriate comments, is impulsive in their actions or has angry outbursts. It is not uncommon that child siblings become the object of negative comments, lose friends and are subjected to teasing or bullying.

Coping with these emotions is, in some regards, dependent on the family functioning, i.e. whether the family have become closer or been pulled apart by their circumstances, and whether appropriate support has been available to them. Some parents become much less available to the non-injured sibling after the accident, as they are caring for the injured child, so many siblings have to grow up fast and become relatively independent quickly. Siblings may become closely involved in the care of their injured sibling and feel needed, acquire new skills and abilities, and develop new interests together; this can enhance the relationship and be supportive to family functioning. Whilst there may be associated stresses and distress as a consequence of this, it can also be valuable for the development of a very positive and fulfilling relationship. Some siblings adjust their choices and priorities in life, in anticipation of being required for care responsibilities in the future.

Siblings are often forgotten after brain injury and their needs may be ignored unless specific issues arise in respect to their health. These health issues may or may not be associated with their sibling's brain injury and, unless practitioners working with the injured sibling have an understanding of their situation and what they are coping with, the main issues of concern may not be addressed. Professionals need to attend to the needs of siblings and consider them within the rehabilitation process and family unit.

As with other family members, siblings need to feel heard and have the opportunity and support to express their thoughts and explore their feelings safely and without judgement. The more the family have to cope with, and the more the injured individual has changed, the more likely the whole family, including the siblings, will be affected. As the sibling's mental health and wellbeing is tied in with the general health and functioning of the family, all members appear to need their own support individually as well as in the family unit.

Children

Deidre (an adult looking after her father) commented, 'knowledge is power' and advised, 'ask questions and learn, and keep asking questions until you feel satisfied you have the right answers. If you do not feel happy with the answers, continue asking and do not make decisions unless they feel right'. 'Do whatever needs to be done or ensure others do and do not wish or regret what you could have done'. Deidre acknowledged the need for support and said, 'Take time away and talk to someone'.

The children, Alistair and Beatrix, when asked what they felt would help, said *'Look after yourself'* and acknowledged that *'Time helps to get acceptance'*. The experiences they had during their childhood were highlighted in their recommendations. They stressed how important it was to *'take opportunities for a break away from tense situations'* and *'having activities or hobbies to immerse self in away from the home environment'*. The children noted the benefit of support from family, neighbours, friends or a support group and someone who would be there for them (in this case the case manager), to help defuse tense situations.

Children will be affected by the trauma of seeing the distress of their parent and other family members. They may not know what is happening, especially in the initial stages and early recovery. The children may have to spend long periods with childminders, neighbours or relatives without really knowing what is going on. As would be expected, all children are affected by trauma, but the level of understanding will depend on the age of the child, what they are able to cope with and the changes in family functioning and dynamics over time.

It is essential to listen and understand the childrens' perspectives and what they believe will help. Providing clear, age-specific and (perhaps) pictorial information about brain injury and engaging them in positive approaches and simple routines can help the children feel valued and involved in supporting the non-injured parent, rather than excluded and on the periphery of what is happening.

Children may seek clarity of information relating to their injured relative, as and when they feel ready, and require emotional support at different stages in their life. Parents or professionals may also determine when this support may be required. The timing of interventions will depend on the child's cognitive development with the transitions of changing schools, teenage years, going to college/work, getting married or having children themselves.

Supporting parents who have a brain injury to develop the ability to care for their children (Brown et al., 2015, 2014), and adapt their coping style (Prihadi et al., 2015) have proved successful, as has skilled and specialist social work and brain injury case management intervention (Holloway, 2016, Holloway and Tyrrell, 2016).

Working with professionals

In the contributors' reflections on their experiences, there were many occasions when they did not receive the input, support or understanding from professionals who were assigned to assess or work with them. In the discussions the contributors provided guidance for all professionals working with families who are in similar situations to themselves.

Trust

Laura, whose husband is in a care establishment, highlighted the importance of being able to trust professionals and those caring for their relative with the brain injury. Her feelings of guilt about not looking after her husband on a full-time basis were reduced by knowing he was well cared for and was happy and content enough.

The family members stressed the importance of professionals getting to know about the individual with the brain injury and their family prior to the accident, as this provided the context for everything afterwards. The relatives appreciated the opportunity to tell their story at the right time for them, so their personal feelings and emotions could be recognised and validated. Timing was critical.

Therapeutic alliance

The family members described their reliance on the professionals to support them and the importance of safe and respectful therapeutic relationships. The contributors described how first meetings could feel particularly threatening and asked professionals to remember that the families were new to this experience and struggling with the complexities of what was going on, not only with their relative with the brain injury but and also with everything else, e.g. dealing with the fallout, holding the family together, bringing up children alone amongst so many uncertainties, caring for the partner, managing house and garden, finances, etc. They wanted professionals to be sensitive to their situation, listen to their concerns and to go gently with them.

The contributors acknowledged those professionals who were able to provide comfort and support during periods of distress and grief. They appreciated when the professionals showed that they cared about them, as well as their relative, and gave them positive feedback and validation as to what they said and did. Emotional support was particularly appreciated at times of crisis and change.

The families wanted professionals to listen to them, and not judge them when discussing their own needs and the injured parties' wishes, intentions and preferences. The families expressed the benefits of open and honest communication, using language they understood. Some relatives felt they had to learn a new 'professional' language.

Families appreciated having support from professionals who listened, were available to talk to, were kind and considerate but not overly demanding of their time. They appreciated people who asked if anything could be done to help, even if this support was initially rejected. The families recognised when the professionals got it right and had an understanding of brain injury and the complexities of their situation; as they felt listened to and the professionals avoided coming up with simplistic, unworkable solutions to complex problems. They acknowledged the professionals who spent time with them recognising what they were doing and helping them make sense of and understand what they were seeing and doing with their relative in everyday life. These professionals worked with the family members to enable them find ways of coping with the situation to support their injured relative over time.

Therefore in order to begin to establish a rapport with family members, the professional needs to gain a perspective of the family member's situation, hear their story and appreciate the stresses they have been through. Listening and hearing without judgement, gently encouraging an elaboration of issues, when appropriate, will allow family members the time to take a wider perspective and explore options that relieve the burden of care, or alternatively improve the quality of life for the injured individual. There are no easy, quick fixes; it is important to be honest and realistic about the future, but also allow hope for small changes to occur over time. Maintaining a degree of gentle contact/communication (without pressure) over time can go a long way to help families feel they are not alone and someone else cares and is thinking of them.

Consistent and knowledgeable support

The contributors valued the skilled and knowledgeable people working alongside them who could guide and support them long-term, from the start of their journey and through the many challenges they faced following the accident. This background support meant that over time, if they did not know what to do, they knew somebody that could appreciate their situation, understood where they were coming from and were there for them. They believed that having this degree of understanding and support afforded a measure of protection, in respect of their own health, and increased their resilience to cope with the long-term care and rehabilitation of their relative.

Communication

The parents highlighted the importance of open and transparent communication to enable everyone to work together collaboratively. One of the parents said, *'Communicate in a way so others can hear what you need to say but also hear what is being said to you'*. Clear and open communication is necessary. Developing a communication style, like motivational interviewing, which is collaborative and facilitative, provides a supportive environment and the 'space' to support the family to make decisions. This style contrasts with the usual 'consultative' one-way interaction style where instructions or guidance is given, albeit with the best of intentions. People are more likely to adopt new approaches when they feel part of the decision-making process. It is easy for professionals to inadvertently confront families' sensitivities at inappropriate times when they are under great pressure. Such poorly-timed confrontations will negatively impact on the therapeutic relationship. Relevant to these issues is Dan (see Chapter 8) and his description of how the team around his son needed to assimilate into his family to enable this trusting and equal relationship to develop. The professionals have as much to learn as the family do.

Working collaboratively

Laura recommended, *'fight for what you believe in and do not be coerced into making any decisions that you don't feel comfortable with'*. *'Always go with your gut instinct, as that is generally the right one to go with. Do not overthink or worry what others may say. Or regret it later'*.

In the hospital and rehabilitation settings, families need to be involved in their relative's rehabilitation and care. Being encouraged how to do even small tasks can provide relatives with the feeling that they have a role in their relative's recovery, and helps prepare them for (potentially) a care-giving role when their relative is discharged home. Family engagement in rehabilitation is recommended, as this leads to better outcomes (Foster et al., 2012).

Rehabilitation has to be relevant to the individual with the brain injury and their family. Professionals often focus on the injured person in isolation and out of their natural context. Too often treatment in hospital or rehabilitation units places little emphasis on the wider family which could help the professionals understand and support situations in the real world.

The contributors stated the good professionals realised the importance of working together and acknowledged their role and contributions. They felt validated when involved in the process of shared goals and the planning and decision-making for their relative's rehabilitation. As the most consistent people involved in the injured relatives' day-to-day life, they needed to be included in the rehabilitation process. Without the engagement and support of the family in rehabilitation, the injured individual's engagement in rehabilitation may be less than optimal.

Parents highlighted the importance of everyone working together and having agreed outcomes. They considered this was not only likely to create a more effective rehabilitation and care package for the injured relative, but also helped them, as parents, cope with the challenges they were presented with and strengthened the relationships between all concerned. One of the parents gave the mantras, '*set your aspirations high, never stop working for the best outcome*', '*learn from each other*' and '*have patience. It takes time*'.

Families know their relative better than anyone else, and provide invaluable observations and insights about the individual before and after any accident, their strengths and weakness, and what might promote or serve as a barrier within any rehabilitation programme. The way forward lies in respect, active collaboration and engagement in the rehabilitation process by all parties, whilst appreciating the grief and losses incurred by the injured individual and all members of the family.

Integrating and supporting family members in the design and provision of therapy in the home setting can facilitate positive outcomes. Involving the family as active members of the rehabilitation team helps not only in the education of families but also adds to the specificity and consistency of any treatment programme. Having interventions planned and implemented in the family home (where possible), at a time that is convenient and manageable for the family is important. It provides opportunities for the individual with brain injury and their family members to learn dynamically and collaboratively with members of the rehabilitation team (psychologists and therapists). This approach has been shown to be effective in improving memory and managing problem behaviours (McKinlay and Hickox, 1988) but it does not necessarily reduce the burden and stress experienced by family members (Carnevale, 2002 and 2006). Although family involvement may be more readily accepted as a concept, in reality input is often limited by logistics, previously-established patterns of working, attitudes and funding, amongst other variables (Shaw, 1990, Levack, 2009, Webster, 1999). Despite knowing that family perceptions and functioning positively affect rehabilitation outcome, and of the need to include both the brain injured person and family in rehabilitation, little seems to have been accomplished to formulate and set up the systems and the professional training necessary to establish this.

Coordination and teamwork

There are major problems in our systems of services for those people with brain injury whose needs do not fall conveniently within the boundaries of a single agency or professional group.

The coordination of rehabilitation programmes for individuals with brain injury can be complex due to the unique presentation of a variety of symptoms and disabilities, the numerous medical, therapeutic and social care specialists required to provide guidance, and the available resources. The family can have many people working with them, asking similar questions but working in isolation from each other. This can increase rather than reduce stress.

Having the support of an interdisciplinary team working together with the brain-injured individual and their family on shared goals in rehabilitation can be cost-effective. Opportunities for learning in consistent routines, supporting the transferring and generalising of functional skills in everyday life, potentially enhances positive outcomes. Coordinating the team requires skilled and careful management to ensure the timing for different aspects of the rehabilitation is appropriate, is undertaken at a pace that is manageable and does not place undue stress on those involved.

Some individuals with brain injury and their families have the opportunity to have case managers specialised in brain injury, funded via a solicitor or Continuing Commissioning Group. The case manager can use their specialist knowledge and experience to work with the individual with brain injury and their family, and guide and support them through the tangled, complex web of resources to establish what is required and coordinate the rehabilitation and support to achieve a lifestyle and quality of life they wish for. This can include a return to increased independence, fulfilment of roles and relationships, socialising with others and integration into work, vocational or leisure activities. This can be a short or long-term intervention depending on the needs of the individual with brain injury and their families over time.

The expert companion: support over time

Do not walk in front of me – I may not follow
Do not walk behind me – I may not lead
Walk beside me and be my friend.

(Anon.)

Grace described how she found having a consistent professional working with her brother and the family over a long period of time invaluable, as this enabled her to know there was someone whom they trusted, who knew them and could be available for support as and when required.

Appropriate skilled support can help structure and integrate the traumatic experience, so it is better understood and easier to contend with. The nature of the ambiguity of the losses suffered by relatives and the lack of community understanding of the experience serves to isolate the relative and provides no clear and straightforward path to a solution. The relatives' experience of trauma is secondary, but they are affected by the trauma that has occurred to their relative. The relatives' sense of what has worked for them resonated with our understanding of the concept of the 'expert companion', a humanising co-traveller on a transformative journey to discover a new reality and seek to accommodate (even if not to accept or adjust to) life post-ABI (Calhoun and Tedeschi, 2013). The companion recognises the individuality, not the homogeneity, of the affected parties and, in so doing, the approach facilitates meaning, creates a sense of agency, acknowledges uniqueness and supports the idea that the person is engaged in navigating a life journey. The approach encourages a sense of closeness so that the distressed individuals who feel hopeless are able to feel more empowered (Lundqvist et al., 2002). Kreutzer et al. (2016) stress the need to work with relatives on their sense of ambiguity and to recognise and explicitly understand these feelings, in order to promote emotional recovery. The expert, like the relative, embarks on this life-narrative in the spirit of brainstorming and collaboration, having no preconceptions of where the story will end. For the relative it is like stepping into the unknown and cannot be undertaken in the absence of trust and the time to explore. The expert companion recognises his or her own limitations and is open to changing, learning from the relative-survivor. Clinicians who see themselves as expert companions practise this humility with trauma survivors, because it is all that is really possible under difficult circumstances that have no ready answers (Calhoun and Tedeschi, 2006b).

In our experience as professionals working with families over long periods of time, as evident from the information in the previous chapters, friction can develop between the family members and professionals for a number of different reasons. Being aware of these issues can aid understanding and potentially reduce the issues that arise.

As professionals, when we encounter families for the first time, we are thrust into the lives of others who we know nothing about. We may see incredible strength and resilience, we may see optimism and resourcefulness, we may see fear, anger, denial or chaos, or all of these things at the same time. We may experience rejection, we may feel blamed or overly responsible, and we may struggle to see light at the end of the tunnel. If there is one message from this book it is this: that the family is probably doing the best it can with the resources available. If we remember this, we are better placed to start supporting the long and endless journey on which family members find themselves.

References

Andersson, K., Bellon, M., & Walker, R. 2016. Parents' experiences of their child's return to school following acquired brain injury (ABI): a systematic review of qualitative studies. *Brain Injury*, 30, 829–838.

Bond, E., Fraeger, C.R.L., Mandleco, B., & Donnelly, M. 2003. Needs of family members of patients with severe traumatic brain injury. *Critical Care Nurse*, 23–24, 63–71.

Brooks, D.N., & McKinlay, W. 1983. Personality and behavioural change after severe blunt head injury: a relative's view. *J Neurol Neurosurg Psychiatry*, 46, 336–344.

Brown, F. L., Whittingham, K., Boyd, R.N., Mckinlay, L., & Sofronoff, K. 2014. Improving child and parenting outcomes following paediatric acquired brain injury: a randomised controlled trial of Stepping Stones Triple P plus Acceptance and Commitment Therapy. *J Child Psychol Psychiatry Allied Discip*, 55, 1172–1183.

Brown, F.L., Whittingham, K., Boyd, R.N., Mckinlay, L., & Sofronoff, K. 2015. Does Stepping Stones Triple P plus Acceptance and Commitment Therapy improve parent, couple, and family adjustment following paediatric acquired brain injury? A randomised controlled trial. *Behav Res Ther*, 73, 58–66.

Butera-Prinzi, F., Charles, N., & Story, K. 2014. Narrative family therapy and group work for families living with acquired brain injury. *Australian and New Zealand Journal of Family Therapy*, 35, 81–99.

Calhoun, L., & Tedeschi, R. 2006a. Expert companions: posttraumatic growth in clinical practice. In: *Handbook of posttraumatic growth: research and practice* (Calhoun, L., & Tedeschi, R., eds). Mahwah, NJ: Lawrence Erlbaum Associates.

Calhoun, L.G., & Tedeschi, R.G. 2006b. *Handbook of posttraumatic growth: research and practice*. Mahwah, NJ: Lawrence Erlbaum Associates.

Calhoun, L.G., & Tedeschi, R.G. 2013. *Posttraumatic growth in clinical practice*. Abingdon and New York: Routledge.

Carnevale, G.J., Anselmi, V., Busichio, K., & Millis, S.R. 2002. Changes in ratings of caregiver burden following a community-based behavior management program for persons with traumatic brain injury. *The Journal of Head Trauma Rehabilitation*, 17(2), 83–95.

Carnevale, G.J., Anselmi, V., Johnston, M.V., Busichio, K., & Walsh, V. 2006. A natural setting behavior management program for persons with acquired brain injury: a randomized controlled trial. *Archives of Physical Medicine and Rehabilitation*, 87(10), 1289–1297.

Ducharme, J.M., Spencer, T., Davidson, A., & Rushford, N. 2002. Errorless compliance training: building a cooperative relationship between parents with brain injury and their oppositional children. *American Journal of Orthopsychiatry*, 72, 585–595.

Easton, A., & Atkin, K. 2011. Medicine and patient narratives. *Social Care and Neurodisability*, 2, 33–41.

Fins, J.J., & Solomon, M.Z. 2001. Communication in intensive care settings: the challenge of futility disputes. *Critical Care Medicine*, 29, N10–N15.

Foster, A.M., Armstrong, J., Buckley, A., Sherry, J., Young, T., Foliaki, S., James-Hohaia, T.M., Theadom, A. & McPherson, K.M. 2012. Encouraging family engagement in the rehabilitation process: a rehabilitation provider's development of support strategies for family members of people with traumatic brain injury. *Disability and Rehabilitation*, 34, 1855–1862.

Holloway, M. 2016. Parenting post-ABI: fostering engagement with services 14 years post-injury: a case study. In: *IBIA conference accepted abstracts* (IBIA, ed.). International Brain Injury Association, Eleventh World Congress on Brain Injury, The Hague, Netherlands.

Holloway, M., & Tyrrell, L. 2016. Acquired brain injury, parenting, social work and rehabilitation: supporting parents to support their children. *Journal of Social Work in Disability and Rehabilitation*, 15(3–4), 234–259.

Junqué, C., Bruna, O., & Mataró, M. 1997. Information needs of the traumatic brain injury patient's family members regarding the consequences of the injury and associated perception of physical, cognitive, emotional and quality of life changes. *Brain Injury*, 11, 251–258.

Kitzinger, C., & Kitzinger, J. 2014. Grief, anger and despair in relatives of severely brain injured patients: responding without pathologising. *Clinical Rehabilitation*, 28, 627–631.

Kreutzer, J.S., Kolakowsky-Hayner, S.A., Demm, S.R., & Meade, M.A. 2002. A structured approach to family intervention after brain injury. *Journal of Head Trauma Rehabilitation*, 17, 349–367.

Kreutzer, J.S., Stejskal, T.M., Ketchum, J.M., Marwitz, J.H., Taylor, L.A., & Menzel, J.C. 2009. A preliminary investigation of the brain injury family intervention: impact on family members. *Brain Injury*, 23, 535–547.

Kreutzer, J.S., Marwitz, J.H., Godwin, E.E., & Arango-Lasprilla, J.C. 2010. Practical approaches to effective family intervention after brain injury. *Journal of Head Trauma Rehabilitation*, 25, 113–120.

Kreutzer, J.S., Mills, A., & Marwitz, J.H. 2016. Ambiguous loss and emotional recovery after traumatic brain injury. *Journal of Family Theory and Review*, 8.

Larøi, F. 2003. The family systems approach to treating families of persons with brain injury: a potential collaboration between family therapist and brain injury professional. *Brain Injury*, 17, 175–187.

Levack, W.M.M., Siegert, R.J., Dean, S.G., & Mcpherson, K.M. 2009. Goal planning for adults with acquired brain injury: how clinicians talk about involving family. *Brain Injury*, 23, 192–202.

Lundqvist, A., Nilstun, T., & Dykes, A.K. 2002. Both empowered and powerless: mothers' experiences of professional care when their newborn dies. *Birth*, 29, 192–199.

McKinlay, W.M. & Hickox, A. 1988. How can families help in the rehabilitation of the head injured? *Journal of Head Trauma Rehabilitation*, 3, 64–72.

Molter, N.C. 1979. Needs of relatives of critically ill patients: a descriptive study. *Heart & Lung*, 8, 332–339.

Neimeyer, R.A. 2001. *Meaning reconstruction and the experience of loss*. Washington, DC: American Psychological Association.

Ponsford, J., Olver, J., Ponsford, M., & Nelms, R. 2003. Long-term adjustment of families following traumatic brain injury where comprehensive rehabilitation has been provided. *Brain Injury*, 17, 453–468.

Prihadi, E.J., Dings, F., & Van Heugten, C.M. 2015. Coping styles of parents of children and adolescents with acquired brain injury in the chronic phase. *J Rehabil Med*, 47, 210–215.

Shaw, L.R. & McMahon, B.T. 1990. Family-staff conflict in the rehabilitation setting: Causes, consequences, and implications. *Brain Injury*, 4, 87–93.

Simpson, G., & Yuen, F. (eds) 2018. *Contemporary perspectives on social work in acquired brain injury*. Abingdon: Routledge.

Todres, L., Galvin, K.T., & Dahlberg, K. 2014. Caring for insiderness: phenomenologically informed insights that can guide practice. *International Journal of Qualitative Studies on Health and Well-being*, 9.

Todres, L., Galvin, K.T., & Holloway, I. 2009. The humanization of healthcare: a value framework for qualitative research. *International Journal of Qualitative Studies on Health and Well-being*, 4, 68–77.

Tyerman, A., King, N., & British Psychological, Society 2008. *Psychological approaches to rehabilitation after traumatic brain injury*. Malden, MA: BPS Blackwell.

Webster, G., Daisley, A., & King, N. 1999. Relationship and family breakdown following acquired brain injury: the role of the rehabilitation team. *Brain Injury*, 13, 593–603.

Chapter 10

In conclusion

All of the relatives who have contributed to this book have expressed their own stories in their own ways and from their different perspectives. Whilst these tales are enlightening, deeply personal and reflective, they are also distressing at times. These narratives also explore the 'meaning of life', in respect of themselves and their loved ones, in how their relationships and dynamics within the family change, and how this is inherent in all they do and how it impacts on their present day and future life.

Contributors noted the unavoidable nature of their involvement with their injured relative and said that the difficulties they faced were not limited to issues that solely related to the brain injury. Post-injury negative changes to behaviour, function and independence necessitate the relatives becoming involved in myriad of different and taxing circumstances, frequently being the injured party's only method of connecting to services or others, including wider family. The fact that participants described their burden of care/support as being unavoidable exacerbates their complex grief and losses. They perceive no alternative but to remain involved despite the impact this has upon their own well-being. Participants note that without their input the brain-injured party's situation would deteriorate and that, in most cases, there was no other person, professional or otherwise, who could and would take over their responsibilities so they felt duty-bound to continue. Relatives undertake this long-term and seemingly unending role whilst dealing with other issues and difficulties and alongside other responsibilities. It is perhaps notable that Dan, Laura and Jeanne all had responsibility for school-aged children at the time of the brain injury; those responsibilities (and others) do not lessen or disappear. Without their sustained involvement it is possible to question what would have happened to Paul, to John and Adam, and how much worse their outcomes would have been.

At times it appears that the difficulties experienced by relatives are exacerbated by formal support services. Contributors experienced very significant difficulties with services in terms of lack of information, lack of specialism, complete lack of provision offered, excessive length of time spent without support, poor attitude or behaviour of staff, lack of brain injury awareness by services, lack of understanding of the difficulties experienced by relatives, services not taking responsibility for the range of needs present, and the added pressure of having to fight to access funding for the services that were available. Laura had to take on funding agencies that she perceived as dismissive and uncaring; Jeanne waited ten years for any form of outside help. Ten years. Ten years during which her and her family's life was torn apart.

Experience of the response given by the wider community, including from family and friends, also frequently exacerbated difficulties owing to a lack of understanding of both the nature of the injury experienced but also of the impact this had upon the relative. Negative experiences of formal and informal support further isolates relatives and maintains the grief and ambiguous loss felt. Relatives noted that even when adequate (or improved) support was achieved, their future lives were still greatly affected by the injury. Dan was able to access funding via litigation that enabled his son to have a bespoke and specialised package of community neuro-rehabilitation. This has manifestly and greatly improved Paul's life. However, Dan still remains very heavily involved in his son's life and care and maintains his sense of responsibility and commitment to his son.

Holding the threads together: curating the narrative of the one you love

The interviews for this book and the research that predated it (Holloway, 2017) lead us to reflect upon the role the loving, committed and involved relative plays in holding together the whole story. Overarching everything it seems, the relative is key to holding the narrative threads of the past, the present and the future. They alone are able to perform this task.

Owing to the nature of the brain injuries suffered by all the relatives of the contributors, the injured person is highly unlikely to be able to accurately describe their pre- and post-accident history in as much detail nor have the ability to project into the future as well as Jeanne, Dan, Laura, Grace, Eliza, Deirdre, Alistair, Beatrix and Christine. This loss is a function of ABI. The relative therefore holds historical information and knowledge that is not cogently held elsewhere. They are witnesses to the shattered narrative and changed identity that severe brain injury brings and, as the only party as closely involved and over a long time frame, they are the only individual to hold this knowledge and maintain historical continuity to this extent. The stories told by the contributors have a clear 'fracture' at the point of injury, one that defines the present and future and sets the pre-injury past aside as a separate time that is not recoverable; it is disconnected. Relatives hold on to this story, guard it and nurture it, and do so out of a sense of complicated love despite the burden and damage that doing so may do to them.

There is an interconnection in family relationships over time – with each family member's life defined by the absence of the injured family member in their previous uninjured state. There is a web of shattered and strained human relationships around the injured family member that potentially impacts on their future life and opportunities. There is the life unlived to consider, a loss that is difficult to define and therefore difficult to grieve for; what would have happened without the ABI? Yet, the impact of this complex trauma on family members is often missed by professionals the family encounters. The importance of this interconnectedness is missed, and with it many opportunities to support, to learn and to understand more.

Professionals are often ill-equipped to respond to a relative's distress and grief, and the emotional pain and hardship experienced could be overwhelming to them if they allowed it in. Services usually focus on the needs of the injured party, without fully appreciating or understanding the impact of this accident on their family. Most services for individuals with brain injury are focused on assessments at discrete times, meaning that most clinicians avoid, or are adrift from, those family members who experience the impact of the injuries as a daily reality. The professionals often do not appear to engage with relatives in a responsive, compassionate way. There are few services that provide individual family support from experienced specialists in the field of brain injury, let alone relatives' groups or sessions for the whole family. Services around the country vary considerably. In the past, consultants in rehabilitation organised regular reviews, so they were part of a system where regular advice and support could be offered. Now in most areas, re-referrals have to be undertaken via their general practitioner. In some areas brain injury case managers or coordinators have been available in the Health Service or Social Services for guidance and support. Their caseloads can be extremely high and overwhelming without the resources required to provide backup rehabilitation and support. Social workers now do not maintain clients on their caseloads for any longer than is perceived necessary, and any referrals back into the system take time and there is inconsistency and a great variability in expertise of people working with them.

The repeated assessments – or constant battles – for funding, whether this is for health or social care or benefits, is a traumatic and overwhelming. This negatively impacts on the relatives and adds unecessary uncertainties, stress and yet another burden to their already shattered lives.

The necessity for professionals to be available for the long haul and walk alongside survivors and their loved ones is paramount. Professionals may need to be oriented to the intimacy of family knowledge and relationships over time, that may not be apparent to strangers or wider family. Professionals may never be able to fully appreciate the pain experienced by families when these bonds have been strained or severed.

The present impacts on future generations; for instance, having safety, security and support promotes emotional resilience and positive relationships for families over time.

All of our contributors are survivors; their survival has been hard fought and at great personal cost; but they have survived. Contained within their stories are clear failings by services and wider society. Underpinning these failures is a basic lack of knowledge of ABI. The effect this has upon individuals and their families. Our contributors gained knowledge over time, knowledge about ABI and about how to navigate services to get the best for their loved ones. They also gained personal experience about what works for them and their injured relative. They have learnt to see broader pictures and, perhaps falteringly and inconsistently, gained some degree of acceptance of what cannot be changed.

We would like to give our heartfelt thanks to all our contributors. Our intention in writing this book is for family members to have the opportunity to say what needs to be said, and for professionals to have an understanding of brain injury, to support families. We, like the families, want their experience to positively change the future of others.

References

Holloway, M. 2017. Acquired brain injury: the lived experience of family members. Doctoral thesis, DSW, University of Sussex.

References

Andersson, K., Bellon, M., & Walker, R. 2016. Parents' experiences of their child's return to school following acquired brain injury (ABI): a systematic review of qualitative studies. *Brain Injury*, 30, 829–838.

Banja, J.D. 2006. Empathy in the physician's pain practice: benefits, barriers and recommendations. *Pain Medicine*, 7, 265–275.

Blake, H. 2014. Caregiver stress in traumatic brain injury. *International Journal of Therapy and Rehabilitation*, 15, 263–271.

Bond, E., Fraeger, C.R.L., Mandleco, B., & Donnelly, M. 2003. Needs of family members of patients with severe traumatic brain injury. *Critical Care Nurse*, 23–24, 63–71.

Boss, P. 1999a. *Ambiguous loss: learning to live with unresolved grief.* Cambridge, MA and London: Harvard University Press.

Boss, P. 1999b. Insights: ambiguous loss: living with frozen grief. *The Harvard Mental Health Letter from Harvard Medical School*, 16, 4–6.

Boss, P. 2000. *Ambiguous loss.* Cambridge, MA: Harvard University Press.

Boss, P. 2006. *Loss, trauma and resilience: therapeutic work with ambiguous loss.* New York: W.W. Norton.

Boss, P. 2010. The trauma and complicated grief of ambiguous loss. *Pastoral Psychology*, 59, 137–145.

Boss, P., & Carnes, D. 2012. The myth of closure. *Family Process*, 51, 456–469.

Brooks, D.N., & McKinlay, W. 1983. Personality and behavioural change after severe blunt head injury: a relative's view. *J Neurol Neurosurg Psychiatry*, 46, 336–344.

Brown, F. L., Whittingham, K., Boyd, R.N., Mckinlay, L., & Sofronoff, K. 2014. Improving child and parenting outcomes following paediatric acquired brain injury: a randomised controlled trial of Stepping Stones Triple P plus Acceptance and Commitment Therapy. *J Child Psychol Psychiatry Allied Discip*, 55, 1172–1183.

Brown, F.L., Whittingham, K., Boyd, R.N., Mckinlay, L., & Sofronoff, K. 2015. Does Stepping Stones Triple P plus Acceptance and Commitment Therapy improve parent, couple, and family adjustment following paediatric acquired brain injury? A randomised controlled trial. *Behav Res Ther*, 73, 58–66.

Butera-Prinzi, F., & Perlesz, A. 2004. Through children's eyes: children's experience of living with a parent with an acquired brain injury. *Brain Injury*, 18, 83–101.

Carnevale, G.J., Anselmi, V., Busichio, K., & Millis, S.R. 2002. Changes in ratings of caregiver burden following a community-based behavior management program for persons with traumatic brain injury. *The Journal of Head Trauma Rehabilitation*, 17(2), 83–95.

Carnevale, G.J., Anselmi, V., Johnston, M.V., Busichio, K., & Walsh, V. 2006. A natural setting behavior management program for persons with acquired brain injury: a randomized controlled trial. *Archives of Physical Medicine and Rehabilitation*, 87(10), 1289–1297.

Caroll, E., & Coetzer, R. 2011. Identity, grief and self-awareness after traumatic brain injury. *Neuropsychological Rehabilitation*, 21(3), 289–305.

Clark-Wilson, J., Giles, G.M., & Baxter, D.M. 2014. Revisiting the neurofunctional approach: conceptualizing the core components for the rehabilitation of everyday living skills. *Brain Injury*, 28(13–14), 1646–1656.

Cooper Evans, S., Alderman, N., Knight, C., & Oddy, M. 2008. Self-esteem as a predictor of psychological distress after severe acquired brain injury: an exploratory study. *Neuropsychological Rehabilitation*, 18(5), 607–626.

Covey, S.R. 2014. *The 7 habits of highly effective families*. New York: St. Martin's Press.

Crosson, B., Poeschel Barco, P., & Velozo, C.A. 1989. Awareness and compensation in post acute head injury rehabilitation. *Journal of Head Trauma Rehabilitation*, 4, 46–54.

Degeneffe, C.E. 2015. Planning for an uncertain future: sibling and parent perspectives on future caregiving for persons with acquired brain injury. *Journal of Rehabilitation*, 81, 5–16.

Degeneffe, C.E. 2016. A clarion call for social work attention: brothers and sisters of persons with acquired brain injury in the United States. *Journal of Social Work in Disability and Rehabilitation*, 1–18.

Degeneffe, C.E, & Olney, M.F. 2010. 'We are the forgotten victims': perspectives of adult siblings of persons with traumatic brain injury. *Brain Injury*, 24 (12), 1416–1427.

De Kloet, A.J., Lambregts, S.A.M., Berger, M.A.M., Van Markus, F., Wolterbeek, R., & Vliet Vlieland, T.P.M. 2015. Family impact of acquired brain injury in children and youth. *Journal of Developmental and Behavioral Pediatrics*, 36, 342–351.

Ducharme, J.M., Spencer, T., Davidson, A., & Rushford, N. 2002. Errorless compliance training: building a cooperative relationship between parents with brain injury and their oppositional children. *American Journal of Orthopsychiatry*, 72, 585–595.

Ergh, T.C., Rapport, L.J., Coleman, R.D., & Hanks, R.A. 2002. Predictors of caregiver and family functioning following traumatic brain injury: social support moderates caregiver distress. *Journal of Head Trauma Rehabilitation*, 17, 155–174.

Fins, J.J. 2015. *Rights come to mind: brain injury, ethics and the struggle for consciousness.* Cambridge: Cambridge University Press.

Fleminger, S. 2008. Long-term psychiatric disorders after traumatic brain injury. *European Journal of Anaesthesiology*, 42(Suppl.), 123–130.

Fleminger, S., & Ponsford, J. 2005. Long term outcome after traumatic brain injury. *British Medical Journal*, 331, 1419–1420.

Fleminger, S., Oliver, D.L., Williams, W., & Evans, J. 2003. The neuropsychiatry of depression after brain injury. *Neuropsychological Rehabilitation*, 13(1–2), 65–87.

Foster, A.M., Armstrong, J., Buckley, A., Sherry, J., Young, T., Foliaki, S., James-Hohaia, T.M., Theadom, A., & McPherson, K.M. 2012. Encouraging family engagement in the rehabilitation process: a rehabilitation provider's development of support strategies for family members of people with traumatic brain injury. *Disability and Rehabilitation*, 34, 1855–1862.

Godwin, E., Chappell, B., & Kreutzer, J. 2014. Relationships after TBI: a grounded research study. *Brain Injury*, 28, 398–413.

Gosling, J., & Oddy, M. 1999. Rearranged marriage: marital relationship after head injury. *Brain Injury*, 13: 785–796.

Gracey, F., & Ownsworth, T. (eds) 2008. The self and identity in rehabilitation. *Neuropsychological Rehabilitation* (Special Issue), 18(5–6).

Hartwell, C. As you are now, so once was I: a reflection on empathy when working with persons with acquired brain injury. www.internationalbra inorg. Houston, TX, USA.

Heary, C., Hogan, D., & Smyth, C. 2004. Parenting a child with acquired brain injury: a qualitative study. *Psychology and Health*, 19, 74–75.

Holloway, M. 2012. Motivational interviewing and acquired brain injury. *Social Care and Neurodisability*, 3: 122–130.

Holloway, M. 2016. Parenting post-ABI: fostering engagement with services 14 years post-injury: a case study. In: *IBIA conference accepted abstracts* (IBIA, ed.). International Brain Injury Association, Eleventh World Congress on Brain Injury, The Hague, Netherlands.

Holloway, M. 2017. Acquired brain injury: the lived experience of family members. Doctoral thesis, DSW, University of Sussex.

Holloway, M., & Tyrrell, L. 2016. Acquired brain injury, parenting, social work and rehabilitation: supporting parents to support their children. *Journal of Social Work in Disability and Rehabilitation*, 15(3–4), 234–259.

Hughes, N., Williams, H., Chitsabesari, P. *et al.* 2015. The prevalence of traumatic brain injury among young offenders in custody: a systematic review. *Journal of Head Trauma Rehabiliation*, 30(2), 94–105.

Jackson, D., Turner-Stokes, L., Murray, J., Leese, M., & Mcpherson, K.M. 2009. Acquired brain injury and dementia: a comparison of carer experiences. *Brain Injury*, 23, 433–444.

Jackson, H.F., & Hague, G. 2013. Social consequences and social solutions: community neurorehabilitation in real social environments. In: *Practical neuropsychological rehabilitation in acquired brain injury* (Newby, G., Coetzer, R. & Daisley, A., eds). London: Karnac Books.

Jenkins, R. 2006. *Social identity*. Abingdon: Routledge.

Jones, L., & Morris, R. 2013. Experiences of adult stroke survivors and their parent carers: a qualitative study. *Clinical Rehabilitation*, 27, 272–280.

Jordan, J., & Linden, M.A. 2013. 'It's like a problem that doesn't exist': the emotional well-being of mothers caring for a child with brain injury. *Brain Injury*, 27, 1063–1072.

Junqué, C., Bruna, O., & Mataró, M. 1997. Information needs of the traumatic brain injury patient's family members regarding the consequences of the injury and associated perception of physical, cognitive, emotional and quality of life changes. *Brain Injury*, 11, 251–258.

Kao, H.F., & Stuifbergen, A.K. 2004. Love and load: the lived experience of the mother–child relationship among young adult traumatic brain-injured survivors. *Journal of the American Association of Neuroscience Nurses*, 36, 73–81.

Kauffman, J. 2002. *Loss of the assumptive world: a theory of traumatic loss*. New York and London: Brunner-Routledge.

Kieffer-Kristensen, R., Teasdale, T.W., & Bilenberg, N. 2011. Post-traumatic stress symptoms and psychological functioning in children of parents with acquired brain injury. *Brain Injury*, 25, 752–760.

Knox, L., & Douglas, J. 2009. Long-term ability to interpret facial expression after traumatic brain injury and its relation to social integration. *Brain and Cognition*, 69, 442–449.

Knox, L., Douglas, J.M., & Bigby, C. 2016. 'I won't be around forever': understanding the decision-making experiences of adults with severe TBI and their parents. *Neuropsychological Rehabilitation*, 26, 236–260.

Kozloff, R. 1987. Network of social support and the outcome from severe head injury. *Journal of Head Trauma Rehabilitation*, 2: 14–23.

Kreutzer, J.S., Kolakowsky-Hayner, S.A., Demm, S.R., & Meade, M.A. 2002. A structured approach to family intervention after brain injury. *Journal of Head Trauma Rehabilitation*, 17, 349–367.

Kreutzer, J.S., Stejskal, T.M., Ketchum, J.M., Marwitz, J.H., Taylor, L.A., & Menzel, J.C. 2009. A preliminary investigation of the brain injury family intervention: impact on family members. *Brain Injury*, 23, 535–547.

Kreutzer, J.S., Marwitz, J.H., Godwin, E.E., & Arango-Lasprilla, J.C. 2010. Practical approaches to effective family intervention after brain injury. *Journal of Head Trauma Rehabilitation*, 25, 113–120.

Larøi, F. 2003. The family systems approach to treating families of persons with brain injury: a potential collaboration between family therapist and brain injury professional. *Brain Injury*, 17, 175–187.

Lefebvre, H., Pelchat, D., & Levert, M. 2007. Interdisciplinary family intervention program: A partnership among health professionals, traumatic brain injury patients and care giving relatives. *Journal of Trauma Nursing*, 14: 100–113.

Levack, W.M.M., Siegert, R.J., Dean, S.G., & Mcpherson, K.M. 2009. Goal planning for adults with acquired brain injury: how clinicians talk about involving family. *Brain Injury*, 23, 192–202.

Levor, K.D., & Jansen, P. 2000. The traumatic onset of disabling injury in a marriage partner: self-reports of the experience by able-bodied spouses. *Social Work*, 36, 193–201.

Lezak, M.D. 1982. The problem of assessing executive functions. *International Journal of Psychology*, 17, 281–297.

Linden, M.A., & Boylan, A.M. 2010. 'To be accepted as normal': public understanding and misconceptions concerning survivors of brain injury. *Brain Injury*, 24, 642–650.

Maitz, F.A., & Sachs, P.P. 1995. Treating families of individuals with traumatic brain injury from a family systems perspective. *Journal of Head Trauma Rehabilitation*, 10: 1–11.

Manchester, D., & Wood, R.L. 2001. Applying cognitive therapy in neurobehavioural rehabilitation. In: *Neurobehavioural disability and social handicap following traumatic brain injury* (Wood, R.L., & McMillan, T.M., eds). Hove: Psychology Press, pp. 157–174.

McKinlay, W.M. & Hickox, A. 1988. How can families help in the rehabilitation of the head injured? *Journal of Head Trauma Rehabilitation*, 3, 64–72.

Miller, W.R., & Rollnick, S. 2002. *Motivational interviewing* (2nd edition). New York: Guilford Press.

Miller, W.R., & Rollnick, S. 2009. Ten things that MI is not. *Behavioural & Cognitive Psychotherapy*, 37, 129–140.

Molter, N.C. 1979. Needs of relatives of critically ill patients: a descriptive study. *Heart & Lung*, 8, 332–339.

Moules, S., & Chandler, B.J. 1999. A study of the health and social needs of carers of traumatically brain injured individuals served by one community rehabilitation team. *Brain Injury*, 13, 983–993.

Moyers, T.B. 2014. The relationship in motivational interviewing. *Psychotherapy*, 51(5), 358–363.

Murphy, A., Huang, H., Montgomery, E.B.Jr., & Turkstra, L. 2015. Conversational turn-taking in adults with acquired brain injury. *Aphasiology*, 29, 151–168.

Owen, F., & Martin, W. 2018. Assessing decision making capacity after brain injury: a phenomenological approach. *Philosophy, Psychiatry & Psychology*, 25(1), 1–19.

Perlesz, A., Kinsella, G., & Crowe, S. 1999. Impact of traumatic brain injury on the family: a critical review. *Rehabilitation Psychology*, 44, 6–35.

Petersen, H., & Sanders, S. 2015. Caregiving and traumatic brain injury: coping with grief and loss. *Health and Social Work*, 40, 325–328. doi:10.1093/hsw/hlv063.

Ponsford, J., Olver, J., Ponsford, M., & Nelms, R. 2003. Long-term adjustment of families following traumatic brain injury where comprehensive rehabilitation has been provided. *Brain Injury*, 17, 453–468.

Prigitano, G.P. 1999. *Principles of neuropsychological rehabilitation*. Oxford: Oxford University Press.

Prigatano, G.P., & Gupta, S. 2006. Friends after traumatic brain injury in children. *Journal of Head Trauma Rehabilitation*, 21, 505–513.

Prigitano, G.P., *et al*. 1986. *Neuropsychological rehabilitation after brain injury.* Baltimore, MD: Johns Hopkins University Press.

Prihadi, E.J., Dings, F., & Van Heugten, C.M. 2015. Coping styles of parents of children and adolescents with acquired brain injury in the chronic phase. *J Rehabil Med*, 47, 210–215.

Report by the Acquired Brain Injury and Mental Capacity Act Interest Group. 2014. *Acquired brain injury and mental capacity: recommendations for action following the House of Lords Select Committee Post-Legislative Scrutiny Report into the Mental Capacity Act.*

Rowlands, A. 2000. Understanding social support and friendship: implications for intervention after acquired brain injury. *Brain Impairment*, 1.

Shaw, L.R., & McMahon, B.T. 1990. Family–staff conflict in the rehabilitation setting: Causes, consequences, and implications. *Brain Injury*, 4, 87–93.

Shorland, J., & Douglas, J.M. 2010. Understanding the role of communication in maintaining and forming friendships following traumatic brain injury. *Brain Injury*, 24, 569–580.

Simpson, G., & Jones, K. 2013. How important is resilience among family members supporting relatives with traumatic brain injury or spinal cord injury? *Clinical Rehabilitation*, 27, 367–377.

Simpson, G., Sabaz, M., & Daher, M. 2013. Prevalence, clinical features, and correlates of inappropriate sexual behavior after traumatic brain injury: a multicenter study. *Journal of Head Trauma Rehabilitation*, 28, 202–210.

Simpson, G.K., & Baguley, I.J. 2012. Prevalence, correlates, mechanisms, and treatment of sexual health problems after traumatic brain injury: a scoping review. *Critical Reviews in Physical and Rehabilitation Medicine*, 24, 1–34.

Skloot, F. 2003. *In the shadow of memory*. Lincoln: University of Nebraska Press.

Summerfield, P. 2011. *Serious case review executive summary in respect of Child H*. North Tyneside: North Tyneside Local Safeguarding Children Board.

Togher, L. 2013. Improving communication for people with brain injury in the 21st century: the value of collaboration. *Brain Impairment*, 14, 130–138.

Togher, L., Mcdonald, S., Tate, R., Rietdijk, R., & Power, E. 2016. The effectiveness of social communication partner training for adults with severe chronic TBI and their families using a measure of perceived communication ability. *NeuroRehabilitation*, 38, 243–255.

Trevena-Peters, J., Ponsford, J., & McKay, A. 2018. Agitated behavior and activities of daily living retraining during posttraumatic amnesia. *The Journal of Head Trauma Rehabilitation*, 33(5), 317–325.

Tyerman, A., King, N., & British Psychological, Society 2008. *Psychological approaches to rehabilitation after traumatic brain injury.* Malden, MA: BPS Blackwell.

Uysal, S., Hibbard, M.R., Robillard, D., Pappadopulos, E., & Jaffe, M. 1998. The effect of parental traumatic brain injury on parenting and child behavior. *Journal of Head Trauma Rehabilitation*, 13, 57–71.

Walsh, F. 2006. *Strengthening family resilience* (2nd edition). New York: Guilford Press.

Webb, D. 1998. A 'revenge' on modern times: notes on traumatic brain injury. *Sociology*, 32, 541–555.

Williams, C., & Wood, R.L. 2013. The impact of alexithymia on relationship quality and satisfaction following traumatic brain injury. *Journal of Head Trauma Rehabilitation*, 28, E21–E30.

Wongvatunyu, S., & Porter, E.J. 2008a. Changes in family life perceived by mothers of young adult TBI survivors. *Journal of Family Nursing*, 14, 314–332.

Wongvatunyu, S., & Porter, E.J. 2008b. Helping young adult children with traumatic brain injury: the life-world of mothers. *Qualitative Health Research*, 18, 1062–1074.

Wood, R.L., & Yurdakul, L.K. 1997. Change in relationship status following traumatic brain injury. *Brain Injury*, 11, 491–501.

Yeates, G., & Daisley, A. 2013. Working with relationships in standard neurorehabilitation practice. In: *Practical neuropsychological rehabilitation in acquired brain injury* (Newby, G., Coetzer, R., & Daisley, A., eds). London: Karnac Books.

Webster, G., Daisley, A., & King, N. 1999. Relationship and family breakdown following acquired brain injury: the role of the rehabilitation team. *Brain Injury*, 13, 593–603.

Index

acceptance 8
acquired brain injury (ABI): enduring nature of 73–74; impact of 4–7; relationships of people with (*See* relationships); *see also* brain injuries
acute treatment 8
ambiguous loss 14–15, 67, 88, 119–120, 154
ambivalence 15
anger 32–33, 37, 50, 57, 95–96, 146
anxiety 10, 13–14, 79, 132, 139, 143
attachment 38–39

best interests 36
brain injuries: acute treatment 8; aggressive behaviours and 50; attitudes of others 97–98, 126–127; causes of 3; deficits (*See* deficits); families acknowledging 47–48; family support for (*See* parents, siblings, spouse/partners); generic information on 139; goal setting with 57; inter-connection in relationships 72–73; life-span approach to services 74; mood shifts and 93, 94; obsessive compulsive disorder 123; psychological connections between people and 74–75; relationships of people with (*See* relationships); sibling's view of 80; socially inappropriate behaviours 57; specificity of information 140; surviving 4; *see also* acquired brain injury (ABI), traumatic experiences

British Association of Brain Injury Case Managers (BABICM) 11
burden of care 13–14, 123, 140–141, 145, 150, 158

capacity 36
Care Commissioning Group (CCG) 66, 71, 135, 153
case managers: early assessments and 27–28; frank discussions with 28–29; helpfulness of 11; need for family inclusion 29; specialising in brain injury 153; value to children 99–100
charitable organisations 70, 74, 126, 139
childhood acquired brain injury 16
children of brain injury parent: abuse and fear of parent 94; advice to other families 104, 111; on attitudes of others 97–98; case managers' value 99–100; changing relationship over time 131–133; compartmentalising home and work life 108; coping strategies 94; employers' lack of sympathy 107; on father's behaviour 93–94; friends, relationship with 96, 98–99, 109; future concerns 103–104; grandparents and 96; guilt and 107; impact on family unit 94, 108–109; impact on personal life 107; leading separate life from parent 99; on leaving injured parent 102–103; litigation process 110; on lost childhood 97;

managing fears 110–111; need for safety 100; perspectives of the accident 93; pre-accident 105; as protector to family members 95; recognising changes in parent 132; rehabilitation and 106; role reversals 95, 128; safety and security for 92, 115, 132; support, benefit of 147–148; taking on adult responsibilities 94–96; trauma, effects of 92; visitation rights of 146
closure 14, 119
cognitive changes 9–10
cognitive impairment: invisibility of 22–23; noticing 26–27, 48; patient unaware of 28; team understanding 29–31
collaborative rehabilitation 151–152
communication 15–16, 23, 64, 125–126, 134–135, 151
community support 56
Continuing Health Care (CHC) 65, 71, 135
coordination of rehabilitation programmes 153
coping 39–40, 71, 115–116, 134–137
crisis see traumatic experiences

decision making: diagnosing problems in 30; in the world 6
deficits: families learning of 49, 116; invisible 5, 9, 118, 125; types of 3–4
Department of Health 74
depression 5, 10, 14, 57, 142–143
despair 142
Different Strokes 70
discharge planning 8–9
disinhibited behaviours 7

embarrassment 86, 121, 124, 146
emotional challenges 121–122
emotion-focused coping 40
emotions 32–33, 50, 69–70, 142, 146–147 see also guilt, loss and grief
empathy 57, 67–68
executive functioning disorders 5–6
executive impairments 5–7
expert companion 154

families: acknowledging trauma 47–48; brain injury research and 12–16; challenges for 5–7; coping and 39–40; duty and responsibility over time 117–118; increasing quality of life 4; roles and responsibilities of 12, 127–133, 143–144; stress and burden on 13–14; support groups for 143; teams engaging with 37–38; unprepared 13; see also children of brain injury parent, parents, siblings, spouse/partners
family adjustment: coping and 39–40; as a process 41
father-son relationship 25, 34, 127–128, 129
feelings see emotions
financial losses 120
frontal lobe injuries 7, 57

grandparents 99, 103, 130, 133
grief see loss and grief
guilt 71, 81, 101, 107, 121, 144

Headway 40, 53–54, 70, 136
hospital discharge 26
House of Lords Select Committee 11

identity 10
identity change, individual's perception of 5
immaturity 51–52, 57
impulsive behaviours 57, 121, 128
inappropriateness 50, 57, 96
independent living 29, 31, 35–36, 45
initiation, diagnosing problems in 30
insight 6–7
interdisciplinary teams 153
invisible deficits 5, 9, 118, 125
isolation, social 7, 57–58, 73

Kids (young carers) 70
knowledge is power 111, 147

litigation process 32, 86, 110, 159
loss and grief: channeling 119; endless 118; feeling of being alone 120; financial losses 120; grieving process 70; lost opportunities 120–121; of normality 121;

ongoing 47–48, 67; personal 4; professionals addressing 55; unresolved 14–15, 34; *see also* ambiguous loss
lost opportunities 120–121

memory deficits 30
Mental Capacity Act 11
mindfulness 142
motivational interviewing 151
Multi-Disciplinary Team (MDT) 29, 36–38, 135

National Service Framework for Long Term (Neurological) Conditions (NSF-LT(n)C) 74
neuropsychology 29–30
normality 121, 142

obsessive behaviours 30–31, 85, 123, 128
Occupational Therapy (OT) 27, 30
OCD, signs of 27
ongoing grief 47–48, 67

parent-child relationship 129
parents: advice to other families 35–37; anger, coping with 32–33, 50; background 24; burden of (*See* burden of care); on changing family dynamics 49–50; changing relationship over time 129–130; collaborative rehabilitation and 152; coping 115; current life with son 24–25; education as key 54; father-son relationship 25, 34, 127–128; frank discussions with case managers 27–29; guilt and shame of (*See* guilt); in hospital 45–46; on immaturity 51–52; independent living trial 31; learning about deficits 49; life after son's accident 25–26; lifelong commitment to their children 23; on loss and grief 55; noticing cognitive problems 26–27; post-accident 49–54; pre-accident 44–45; recovery 46–48; reflections on the future 133; rehabilitation 48; on spouse/partners 33–34; on team's diagnosing

problems 30; on therapy teams 29; *see also* relationships
partners *see* spouse/partners
patience 40
personality changes 9–10
post-injury: challenge recognizing one another 70, 75; quality of life 11; rehabilitation (*See* rehabilitation)
post-traumatic amnesia phase 8
posttraumatic stress disorder 16, 142, 143
pre-accident 24, 44–45, 79–80, 83, 93, 113–114
professionals: addressing loss and grief 55; communication with 125–126, 151; compassion and 73; considering needs of family members 143–148; consistent support 150; getting family 'buy in' 35; ill-equipped to respond 160; knowledgeable support 150; longer-term relationships with 135–136; motivational interviewing 151; offering emotional support 149; rehabilitation 134–135; relationships with families 81, 149–150; support over time 153–154, 161; therapeutic alliance 149–150; trust in 29–31, 35, 39, 121, 124, 135, 149; working with 27–28; working with other professionals 136

quality of life: children increasing parent's 112; coordination of rehabilitation programmes for 153; family members as key to increasing 4; improving 4, 11–12, 150; increased independence and 140; siblings supporting 83, 87, 89–90

recovery 8–10, 46–48
regression 47, 48
rehabilitation 10–12, 29, 35, 48, 64, 134–135, 151–152
relationships: of adults with ABI and their parents 15; breakdown between spouses or partners 15; changing over time 129–133; children of ABI people 16;

developing new 10; father-son 25, 34; forming safe 38; loss of 15–16; with professionals 135–136; sibling 16; with their relative 127–128; *see also* parents

resilience 13–15, 56, 87, 119, 124–125, 142, 150

routines: adapting and developing new 9–10; leading to self-reliance 5

safeguarding children 90, 101

safe relationships 38

safety and security: children of brain injury parent 92, 115, 132; of injured family member 71, 115, 118; loss of 14; need for 138–139; professionals and 100

self-awareness 58

self-concept, changes in 5

self-identity 57

self-regulating behaviour 58

sense of self 141

shame 13–14, 144 *see also* guilt

siblings: advice to other families 83, 90–91; changing relationship over time 131; coping in early stages 116; coping with situation 89; describing relationship 81–82; family functioning and 146–147; hospital discharge 85; impact on family unit 80; independent living trial 87; life before accident 79–80, 84; litigation process 86; mixed emotions of 146–147; overwhelming feelings 81, 86; personal life 90; post-injury 83; professionals attending to needs of 147; relationship with injured sibling 16; role changes 128; role of 87; safeguarding children 90; stress and health issues 87–88; supporting each other 88–89

Simon Says 70

social awareness 103

social isolation 7, 57–58, 73

socially inappropriate behaviours 57

Social Services support 100–101

spouse/partners: on annual assessments 66; background 60–61; changing relationship over time 130–131; conflicting needs of children and injured partner 116; on continuing health care fight 65–66; coping in early stages 116; coping mechanism 71; exploring their feelings 145; feelings of being alone 68; guilt feelings 71; in hospital 61–63; managing the family's emotions 69; at neuro rehabilitation home 65; ongoing grief 67; overwhelming feelings of doing everything 116; professionals working with 145–146; reflections on the future 133–134; in rehab ward 64; on review process 64; separation of 146; stroke survivor 61; in stroke unit 63–64, 116; wanting empathy and support 67–68

statutory health and social care services 10–11

stress: demands and 122–123; on families 13–14; health issues and 87–88; mental health and 141–143

Stroke Association 70

support groups *see* charitable organisations

support services 159, 160–161

task-oriented coping 40

teams *see* Multi-Disciplinary Team (MDT)

therapeutic alliance 58, 149–150

third sector organisations *see* charitable organisations

traumatic brain injuries 7

traumatic experiences: acknowledging 47–48; coping in early stages 115–116; discharge home 116–117; immediate aftermath 25, 45–48, 61–63, 80, 93, 114–115; overwhelming feelings 14, 36, 81, 86, 116

trust: absence of 154; communication creating 125, 151; establishing 90; with grandchildren 103; in others, as a parent 135; in professionals 29–31, 35, 39, 121, 124, 135, 149